This report contains the collective views of an international group of experts and does not necessarily represent the decisions or the stated policy of the United Nations Environment Programme, the International Labour Organisation, or the World Health Organization.

Environmental Health Criteria 109

SUMMARY REPORT ON THE EVALUATION OF SHORT-TERM TESTS FOR CARCINOGENS (COLLABORATIVE STUDY ON *IN VIVO* TESTS)

Published under the joint sponsorship of
the United Nations Environment Programme,
the International Labour Organisation,
and the World Health Organization

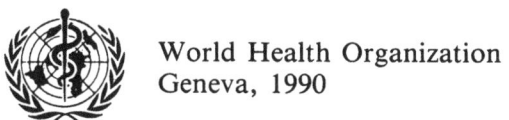

World Health Organization
Geneva, 1990

The **International Programme on Chemical Safety (IPCS)** is a joint venture of the United Nations Environment Programme, the International Labour Organisation, and the World Health Organization. The main objective of the IPCS is to carry out and disseminate evaluations of the effects of chemicals on human health and the quality of the environment. Supporting activities include the development of epidemiological, experimental laboratory, and risk-assessment methods that could produce internationally comparable results, and the development of manpower in the field of toxicology. Other activities carried out by the IPCS include the development of know-how for coping with chemical accidents, coordination of laboratory testing and epidemiological studies, and promotion of research on the mechanisms of the biological action of chemicals.

WHO Library Cataloguing in Publication Data

Summary report on the evaluation of short-term tests for
　　carcinogens : (collaborative study on *in vivo* tests).

　(Environmental health criteria ; 109)

　　1. Carcinogens - analysis　2. Mutagens - analysis
　　3. Mutagenicity tests　　　4. Evaluation studies　　I. Series

　　ISBN 92 4 157109 8　　　(NLM Classification: QZ 202)
　　ISSN 0250-863X

© World Health Organization 1990

Publications of the World Health Organization enjoy copyright protection in accordance with the provisions of Protocol 2 of the Universal Copyright Convention. For rights of reproduction or translation of WHO publications, in part or *in toto,* application should be made to the Office of Publications, World Health Organization, Geneva, Switzerland. The World Health Organization welcomes such applications.

　　The designations employed and the presentation of the material in this publication do not imply the expression of any opinion whatsoever on the part of the Secretariat of the World Health Organization concerning the legal status of any country, territory, city, or area or of its authorities, or concerning the delimitation of its frontiers or boundaries.

　　The mention of specific companies or of certain manufacturers' products does not imply that they are endorsed or recommended by the World Health Organization in preference to others of a similar nature that are not mentioned. Errors and omissions excepted, the names of proprietary products are distinguished by initial capital letters.

Printed in Finland
90/8449 — Vammala — 5000

CONTENTS

	SYNOPSIS	14
1.	INTRODUCTION	18
2.	THE COLLABORATIVE STUDY ON SHORT-TERM *IN VIVO* TESTS FOR MUTAGENS AND CARCINOGENS (CSSTT/2) 1983-85	22
3.	OVERALL AIMS OF THE STUDY AND CRITERIA FOR THE SELECTION OF AN APPROPRIATE SHORT-TERM *IN VIVO* TEST	26

    3.1 The use of short-term tests for the primary identification of genotoxic chemicals   26
    3.2 The use of short term *in vivo* assays for assessing the hazard associated with exposure to *in vitro* genotoxins   27
    3.3 The role of short-term *in vitro* tests in research into the mechanisms of cancer   28
    3.4 Assays for the detection of germ cell mutagens   29

4.	CRITERIA FOR THE SELECTION OF THE FOUR TEST CHEMICALS	30

    4.1 Activity of the four test chemicals in short-term *in vitro* tests   30
    4.2 Summary of carcinogenicity data on the test chemicals   31

5.	SOURCE AND PURITY OF THE TEST CHEMICALS	33
6.	SHORT-TERM *IN VIVO* ASSAYS	34

    6.1 Cytogenetic assays   34
    6.2 Assays in rodent liver cells   36
    6.3 Miscellaneous assays   37
    6.4 The mouse spot test   39
    6.5 Mammalian germ cell studies   39
    6.6 Drosophila assays   40

7.	**RESULTS**	41
	7.1 Benzo[a]pyrene and pyrene	41
	7.1.1 Cytogenetic studies	41
	7.1.2 Liver-specific assays	44
	7.1.3 Miscellaneous assays	46
	7.1.4 Mouse spot tests	47
	7.1.5 Mammalian germ cell assays	48
	7.1.6 Drosophila assays	48
	7.2 2-Acetylaminofluorene and 4-acetylaminofluorene	48
	7.2.1 Cytogenetic studies	48
	7.2.2 Liver-specific assays	49
	7.2.3 Miscellaneous assays	51
	7.2.4 Mouse spot tests	52
	7.2.5 Mammalian germ cell assays	52
	7.2.6 Drosophila assays	53
	7.3 Summary of the *in vivo* genotoxicity of the four chemicals	53
8.	**ASSESSMENT OF THE PERFORMANCE OF THE ASSAYS**	56
	8.1 Cytogenetic assays	62
	8.1.1 Chromosome aberrations	62
	8.1.2 Micronuclei	63
	8.1.3 Sister chromatid exchange	64
	8.2 Liver assays	66
	8.2.1 Initiation and promotion	66
	8.2.2 Unscheduled DNA synthesis and S-phase analysis	67
	8.2.3 DNA strand breaks	69
	8.2.4 Cytogenetics	69
	8.3 Miscellaneous assays	70
	8.3.1 Specific carcinogenicity assays	70
	8.3.2 Supplementary assays	70
	8.3.3 Immunotoxicity assays	72
	8.3.4 Host-mediated assays and urine mutagenicity tests	73
	8.4 Mouse spot tests	73
	8.5 Assays in mammalian germ cells	74
	8.5.1 Dominant lethal and unscheduled DNA synthesis assay	74
	8.5.2 Sperm abnormality tests	75

	8.6 Drosophila assays	75
9.	SELECTION OF THE MOST EFFECTIVE *IN VIVO* ASSAYS IN RELATION TO THEIR PERFORMANCE	77
	9.1 Assays that are not considered appropriate for routine *in vivo* testing of chemicals for genotoxic activity	77
	9.2 Assays that satisfy some or all of the criteria for an acceptable *in vivo* short-term test	78
	9.2.1 Assays currently in general use	78
	9.2.2 Assays that show promise for future development	80
	9.3 The detection of germ cell mutagens	81
	9.4 Influence of route of administration of the test chemicals	82
10.	CONCLUSIONS	83
	REFERENCES	86
	ETUDE COLLECTIVE POUR L'EVALUATION ET LA VALIDATION DES EPREUVES DE COURTE DUREE RELATIVES AUX CANCEROGENES	88
	ESTUDIO EN COLABORACION SOBRE EVALUACION Y COMPROBACION DE PRUEBAS A CORTO PLAZO PARA SUSTANCIAS CARCINOGENAS	93

PARTICIPANTS IN THE COLLABORATIVE STUDY

Dr I. Adler, Mammalian Genetics Institute, Association for Radiation and Environmental Research, Neuherberg, Federal Republic of Germany

Dr R. Albanese, Pharmaceuticals Division, Imperial Chemical Industries PLC, Macclesfield, Cheshire, England

Dr J.W. Allen, Genetic Toxicology Division, US Environmental Protection Agency, Research Triangle Park, North Carolina, USA

Dr J.A. Allen, Department of Mutagenesis and Cell Biology, Huntingdon Research Centre Ltd., Huntingdon, Cambridgeshire, England

Dr O. Andersen, Odense University, Institute of Community Health, Department of Environmental Medicine, Odense, Denmark

Dr D. Anderson, British Industrial Biological Research Association, Carshalton, Surrey, United Kingdom

Dr J. Arany, Institut d'Hygiène et d'Epidémiologie, Brussels, Belgium

Dr J. Ashby, Central Toxicology Laboratory, Imperial Chemical Industries PLC, Macclesfield, Cheshire, United Kingdom

Dr R.A. Baan, Medical Biological Laboratory TNO, Rijswijk, Netherlands

Dr P. Bannasch, Cytopathology Department, Institute of Experimental Pathology, German Cancer Research Centre, Heidelberg, Federal Republic of Germany

Dr G.C. Becking, International Programme on Chemical Safety, World Health Organization, Research Triangle Park, North Carolina, USA

Dr B. Beije, Department of Genetic and Cellular Toxicology, Wallenberg Laboratory, Stockholm University, Stockholm, Sweden

Dr J. Benes, Institute of Nuclear Biology and Radiochemistry, Prague, Czechoslovakia

Dr E. Bermudez, Department of Genetic Toxicology, Chemical Industry Institute of Toxicology, Research Triangle Park, North Carolina, USA

Dr H.C. Birnboim, Department of Experimental Oncology, Ottawa Regional Cancer Centre, Ottawa, Ontario, Canada

Dr J.B. Bishop, Cellular and Genetic Toxicology Branch, Toxicology Research and Testing Program, National Institute of Environmental Health Sciences, Research Triangle Park, North Carolina, USA

Dr D.H. Blakey, Mutagenesis Section, Environmental Health Centre, Department of National Health and Welfare, Tunney's Pasture, Ottawa, Ontario, Canada

Dr R. Braum, Central Institute for Genetics and for Research on Cultivated Plants, Academy of Science of the German Democratic Republic, Gatersleben, German Democratic Republic

Dr G. Bronzetti, National Research Council, Institute of Mutagenesis and Differentiation, Pisa, Italy

Dr B.E. Butterworth, Chemical Industry Institute of Toxicology, Research Triangle Park, North Carolina, USA

Dr P.S. Chauhan, Bio-Medical Group, Bhabha Atomic Research Centre, Bombay, India

Dr I. Chouroulinkov, Unité de Cancérogénèse Expérimentale et de Toxicologie Génétique (E.R. 304) I.R.S.C.-C.N.R.S., Villejuif, France

Dr M.G. Clare, Shell Research Ltd, Sittingbourne, Kent, United Kingdom

Dr R.D. Combes, School of Biological Sciences, Portsmouth Polytechnic, Portsmouth, United Kingdom

Dr C. Coton, Mammalian Genetics Laboratory, Department of Biology, European Nuclear Centre, Mol, Belgium

Dr R. Crebelli, Higher Institute of Health, Viale Regina Elena, Rome, Italy

Dr B.J. Dean, Upchurch, Sittingbourne, Kent, United Kingdom

Dr G.M. Decad, Department of Materials Toxicology, IBM Corporation, San Jose, California, USA

Dr F.J. de Serres, National Institute of Environmental Health Sciences, Research Triangle Park, North Carolina, USA

Dr D.J. Doolittle, Toxicology Research, Bowman Gray Technical Center, R.J. Reynolds Co., Winston-Salem, North Carolina, USA

Dr U.H. Ehling, Mammalian Genetics Institute, Association for Radiation and Environmental Research, Neuherberg, Federal Republic of Germany

Dr B.M. Elliott, Genetic Toxicology Section, Imperial Chemical Industries PLC, Macclesfield, Cheshire, United Kingdom

Dr R. Fahrig, Fraunhofer Institute for Research on Toxicology and Aerosols, Hannover, Federal Republic of Germany

Dr R. Forster, Life Science Research, Rome Toxicology Centre, Pomezia, Rome, Italy

Dr K. Fujikawa, Drug Safety Evaluation Laboratories, Central Research Division, Takeda Chemical Industries Ltd, Osaka, Japan

Dr C. Furihata, Department of Molecular Oncology, Institute of Medical Science, University of Tokyo, Tokyo, Japan

Dr S.M. Galloway, Merck Sharp & Dohme Research Laboratories, West Point, Pennsylvania, USA

Dr W.M. Generoso, Biology Division, Oak Ridge National Laboratory, Oak Ridge, Tennessee, USA

Dr H.P. Glauert, McArdle Laboratory for Cancer Research, University of Wisconsin, Madison, Wisconsin, USA

Dr U. Graf, Toxicology Institute, Zurich Federal Polytechnic and University, Zurich, Switzerland

Dr B.L. Harper, Division of Environmental Toxicology, University of Texas Medical Branch, Galveston, Texas, USA

Dr G.G. Hatch, Toxicology Division, Northrop Services Inc., Environmental Sciences, Research Triangle Park, North Carolina, USA

Dr M. Hayashi, Biological Safety Research Centre, National Institute of Hygienic Sciences, Tokyo 158, Japan

Dr R.M. Hicks, School of Pathology, Middlesex Hospital Medical School, London, United Kingdom

Dr J.M. Hunt, Department of Pathology and Laboratory Medicine, University of Texas Medical School, Houston, Texas, USA

Dr N. Inui, Biological Research Centre, Japan Tobacco Inc., Kanagawa, Japan

Dr M. Ishidate, Jr., Biological Safety Research Centre, National Institute of Hygienic Sciences, Tokyo, Japan

Dr V.I. Ivanov, Institute of Medical Genetics, Academy of Medical Sciences, Moscow, USSR

Dr J.C. Jensen, National Food Institute, Institute of Toxicology, Copenhagen, Denmark

Dr D. Jenssen, Department of Genetic Toxicology, Wallenberg Laboratory, University of Stockholm, Stockholm, Sweden

Dr B.J. Kilbey, Institute of Animal Genetics, University of Edinburgh, Edinburgh, United Kingdom

Dr I. Kimber, Central Toxicology Laboratory, Imperial Chemical Industries PLC, Macclesfield, Cheshire, United Kingdom

Dr U. Kliesch, Mammalian Genetics Institute, Association for Radiation and Environmental Research, Neuherberg, Federal Republic of Germany

Dr A.D. Kligerman, Environmental Health Research and Testing Inc., Research Triangle Park, North Carolina, USA

Dr D. Kornbrust, Merck Sharp & Dohme Research Laboratories, Department of Safety Assessment, West Point, Pennsylvania, USA

Dr C. Lasne, Unité de Cancérogénèse Expérimentale et de Toxicologie Génétique (ER-304) I.R.S.C.-C.N.R.S., Villejuif, France

Dr A. Léonard, Mammalian Genetics Laboratory, Department of Biology, European Nuclear Centre, Mol, Belgium

Dr C.A. Luke, Medical Department, Brookhaven National Laboratory, Upton, New York, USA

Dr J.T. MacGregor, US Department of Agriculture, Western Regional Research Center, Berkeley, California, USA

Dr A.M. Malashenko, Scientific Research Laboratory of Experimental Biological Models of the Academy of Medical Sciences of the USSR, Moscow Region, USSR

Dr C. Malaveille, International Agency for Research on Cancer, Lyon, France

Dr B.H. Margolin, Biometry and Risk Assessment Program, National Institute of Environmental Health Sciences, Research Triangle Park, North Carolina, USA

Dr D. McGregor, Developmental Toxicology, Inveresk Research International Ltd, Musselburgh, United Kingdom

Dr A.L. Meyer, Shell Research Ltd, Sittingbourne, Kent, United Kingdom

Dr J.C. Mirsalis, Cellular and Genetic Toxicology Department, SRI International, Menlo Park, California, USA

Dr N. Nashed, Johann Wolfgang Goethe-Universität, Frankfurt am Main, Federal Republic of Germany

Dr S.B. Neal, Toxicology Division, Lilly Research Laboratory, Greenfield, Indiana, USA

Dr A. Neuhäuser-Klaus, Mammalian Genetics Institute, Association for Radiation and Environmental Research, Neuherberg, Federal Republic of Germany

Dr D.A. Pagano, Cellular and Genetic Toxicology Branch, Toxicology Research and Testing Program, National Institute of Environmental Health Sciences, Research Triangle Park, North Carolina, USA

Dr F. Palitti, Evolutionary Genetics Centre of the National Research Council, Genetics and Molecular Biology Department, University City, Rome, Italy

Dr S. Parodi, Chemical Carcinogenesis Laboratory, National Cancer Research Institute, Genoa, Italy

Dr M. Pereira, Health Effects Research Laboratory, US Environmental Protection Agency, Cincinnati, Ohio, USA

Dr J. Pot-Deprun, Unité de Cancérogénèse Expérimentale et Toxicologie Génétique (ER-304) I.R.S.C.- C.N.R.S. Laboratoires de Recherche Appliquée sur le Cancer, Villejuif, France

Dr G.S. Probst, Toxicology Division, Lilly Research Laboratories, Greenfield, Indiana, USA

Dr C. Ramel, Wallenberg Laboratory, University of Stockholm, Stockholm, Sweden

Dr K. Randerath, Baylor College of Medicine, Department of Pharmacology, Houston, Texas, USA

Dr H.S. Rosenkranz, Department of Environmental Health Sciences, Case Western Reserve University, Cleveland, Ohio, USA

Dr P. Russo, National Cancer Research Institute, Genoa, Italy

Dr M.F. Salamone, Moe-Biohazard Laboratory, Rexdale, Ontario, Canada

Dr C.B. Salocks, Department of Materials Toxicology, IBM Corporation, San Jose, California, USA

Dr J. Schöneich, Central Institute for Genetics and for Research on Cultivated Plants, Academy of Science of the German Democratic Republic, Gatersleben, German Democratic Republic

Dr A.G. Searle, Medical Research Council Radiobiology Unit, Harwell, Didcot, United Kingdom

Dr G.A Sega, Biology Division, Oak Ridge National Laboratory, Oak Ridge, Tennessee, USA

Dr M.D. Shelby, Cellular and Genetic Toxicology Branch, Toxicology Research and Testing Program, National Institute of Environmental Health Sciences, Research Triangle Park, North Carolina, USA

Dr H. Shibuya, Laboratory of Genetic Toxicology, Hatano Research Institute, Food and Drug Safety Center, Kanagawa, Japan

Dr T. Shibuya, Laboratory of Genetics, Hatano Research Institute, Food and Drug Safety Center, Kanagawa, Japan

Dr R.H. Stevens, Radiation Research Laboratory, Department of Radiation, University of Iowa, Iowa, USA

Dr G.D. Stoner, Department of Pathology, Medical College of Ohio, Toledo, Ohio, USA

Dr J.A. Styles, Central Toxicology Laboratory, Imperial Chemical Industries PLC, Macclesfield, Cheshire, United Kingdom

Dr K.E. Suter, Preclinical Research, Toxicology Department, Sandoz Limited, Basel, Switzerland

Dr A. D. Tates, Department of Radiation Genetics and Chemical Mutagenesis, State University of Leiden, Leiden, Netherlands

Dr R.R. Tice, Medical Department, Brookhaven National Laboratory, Upton, New York, USA

Dr H. Tsuda, First Department of Pathology, Nagoya City, University Medical School, Nagoya, Japan

Dr R. Valencia, Department of Zoology, University of Wisconsin, Zoology Research Building, Madison, Wisconsin, USA

Dr A. Vlachos, Haskell Laboratory for Toxicology and Industrial Medicine, E.I. Du Pont de Nemours & Co. Inc., Newark, Delaware, USA

Dr E.W. Vogel, Department of Radiation Genetics and Chemical Mutagenesis, State University of Leiden, Leiden, Netherlands

Dr P.A. Watkins, Pharmaceuticals Division, Imperial Chemical Industries PLC, Macclesfield, Cheshire, United Kingdom

Dr G.A. Wickramaratne, Central Toxicology Laboratory, Imperial Chemical Industries PLC, Macclesfield, Cheshire, United Kingdom

Dr D. Wild, Pharmacology and Toxicology Institute, Würzburg University, Würzburg, Federal Republic of Germany

Dr P.K. Working, Department of Genetic Toxicology, Chemical Industry Institute of Toxicology, Research Triangle Park, North Carolina, USA

Dr V.S. Zhurkov, A. N. Sysin Institute of General and Environmental Hygiene, Moscow, USSR

NOTE TO READERS OF THE CRITERIA DOCUMENTS

Every effort has been made to present information in the criteria documents as accurately as possible without unduly delaying their publication. In the interest of all users of the environmental health criteria documents, readers are kindly requested to communicate any errors that may have occurred to the Manager of the International Programme on Chemical Safety, World Health Organization, Geneva, Switzerland, in order that they may be included in corrigenda, which will appear in subsequent volumes.

ABBREVIATIONS

AAF	Acetylaminofluorene
BP	Benzo[a]pyrene
CSSTT/1	Collaborative study on short-term tests for genotoxicity and carcinogenicity
CSSTT/2	Collaborative study on short-term *in vivo* tests for mutagens and carcinogens
GGT	Gamma-glutamyltranspeptidase
IPESTTC	International Collaborative Programme for the Evaluation of Short-Term Tests for Carcinogens
NK	Natural killer
PYR	Pyrene
SCE	Sister chromatid exchange
SSB	Single strand breaks
UDS	Unscheduled DNA synthesis

SYNOPSIS

THE INTERNATIONAL PROGRAMME ON CHEMICAL SAFETY (IPCS) COLLABORATIVE STUDY ON THE ASSESSMENT AND VALIDATION OF SHORT-TERM TESTS FOR CARCINOGENS.

The first part of this project, dealing with *in vitro* studies, was published in 1985 (Ashby et al., 1985) and was summarized in Environmental Health Criteria 47 (WHO, 1985). The second part, which is the subject of this report, was published in 1988 (Ashby et al., 1988a).

The need for inter-laboratory collaborative studies on an international scale arose from the necessity to investigate the value of short-term tests for detecting mutagenic and carcinogenic chemicals. Short-term assays were proposed as alternatives or supplementary procedures to traditional long-term rodent bioassays. Concern about the choice of short-term tests and their reliability and sensitivity led to the instigation of the first major international collaborative exercise, the International Collaborative Programme for the Evaluation of Short-Term Tests for Carcinogens (IPESTTC) (de Serres & Ashby, 1981). The results of this study confirmed the value of the salmonella mutation test as a reliable and practicable assay for the primary identification of carcinogens and mutagens. It was also observed that, in the salmonella test, some known rodent carcinogens were either not detected or only detected with considerable difficulty. Several other assays represented in the IPESTTC study were able to detect some of the rodent carcinogens that were negative in the salmonella assay. The supporting data base was too small, however, to permit the recommendation of an assay that would complement the salmonella mutation test.

It was apparent, from the results of the IPESTTC study, that a further collaborative exercise would be required to establish a) the most effective combination of *in vitro* assays for primary screening of chemicals for genotoxic activity and b) the most useful short-term *in vivo* tests for confirming mammalian genotoxicity and carcinogenic potential. The Collaborative Study on the Assessment and Validation of Short-Term Tests for Genotoxicity and Carcinogenicity (CSSTT) was proposed by the International Programme on Chemical Safety (IPCS) and the National Institute of Environmental Health Sciences (NIEHS) of the USA (a Participating Institution of the IPCS). Because of the complexity of the organization and the magnitude of the project, it was divided into two discrete studies: the Collaborative Study on Short-Term Tests for Genotoxicity and Carcinogenicity (CSSTT/1) and the Collaborative Study on Short-Term *In Vivo* Tests for Mutagens and Carcinogens (CSSTT/2).

In CSSTT/1, a comprehensive data base was assembled from a wide range of *in vitro* assays conducted with ten carefully selected organic chemicals. These included eight established rodent carcinogens that were either negative or difficult to detect in the salmonella assay and two chemicals that were regarded as non-carcinogenic. Data were evaluated from almost 90 sets of assays conducted by some 60 participating scientists. Four types of assays performed well enough to be considered as possible complementary tests to the salmonella assay. These included tests for chromosomal aberrations, gene mutations and neoplastic transformation in cultured mammalian cells, and an assay for aneuploidy in yeast. With the exception of the chromosomal aberration assay, it was apparent that protocols in general use for these assays required further evaluation before they could be considered fully acceptable.

The major conclusion of the CSSTT/1 study on *in vitro* assays was that the use of chromosomal aberration assays in conjunction with the salmonella mutation test may provide an efficient primary screen for possible new carcinogens.

In the IPESTTC study, seven of the fourteen presumed non-carcinogens gave positive results in many of the *in vitro* assays. The limited *in vivo* data available from that study suggested that these seven chemicals were inactive in *in vivo* short-term tests. The non-carcinogens in two of the carcinogen/non-carcinogen pairs in IPESTTC, i.e. benzo[*a*]pyrene/pyrene (BP/PYR) and 2-acetylamino-fluorene/

Synopsis

4-acetylaminofluorene (2AAF/4AAF), provided good examples of these different responses, and these pairs of chemicals were selected for the *in vivo* part of the collaborative study (CSSTT/2). There was, however, a question mark against the presumed non-carcinogenicity of 4AAF, and a vital part of the study was the initiation of long-term cancer bioassays of 2AAF and 4AAF in rats.

The objective of CSSTT/2, therefore, was to generate a comprehensive data profile from a broad range of short-term *in vivo* tests as a means of understanding how various genetic endpoints in key target tissues respond to chemicals defined as genotoxic *in vitro*. The ultimate goal was to identify which *in vivo* assays could be used to determine the *in vivo* activity of established genotoxins.

Ninety-seven investigators from sixteen countries participated in the *in vivo* project and data were presented from some fifty separate *in vivo* techniques. The results were evaluated at a meeting of investigators held at Cap d'Agde, France, in May 1985. A series of reports were prepared comprising an assessment of each group of assays, summary reports on the germ cell assays and the liver-specific tests, and summary reports on the total data base on each pair of chemicals. Subsequently, an overview of the whole *in vivo* study was prepared in readiness for final publication.

The criteria defining an acceptable short-term *in vivo* test were satisfied by only a small proportion of the assays represented in CSSTT/2. However, the assays included in the study were not limited to those most likely to meet the criteria. Thus, although data were submitted from assays not designed primarily to identify *in vivo* genotoxicity, they provided information on a broad spectrum of biological effects of the four chemicals. Most of the *in vivo* somatic cell assays for genotoxicity discriminated between the two carcinogen/non-carcinogen pairs although, in some cases, weak activity was detected in tests with the non-carcinogens, particularly with 4AAF. The insensitivity of some assays to one or other of the two pairs of chemicals support the concept that negative *in vivo* data should be obtained from at least two assays in different tissues before a chemical can be accepted as non-genotoxic *in vivo*.

The mouse bone marrow micronucleus test was confirmed as a robust, sensitive, and reproducible assay and was recommended for primary *in vivo* testing of *in vitro* genotoxins. The overall performance of the rat liver assay for unscheduled DNA synthesis suggested that it could be complementary to the micronucleus test, although certain aspects of the sensitivity and selectivity of this assay require additional investigation. Some widely advocated assays including the host-mediated and urine mutagenicity assays and tests using drosophila were concluded to be inappropriate for hazard-assessment purposes.

The results of the CSSTT/2 study confirmed that short-term *in vivo* tests have a vital role to play in hazard assessment and that this role is to identify those chemicals, shown to be genotoxic *in vitro*, that are active *in vivo* and, thus, are most likely to present a carcinogenic/mutagenic hazard to mammals, including humans.

1. INTRODUCTION

For many years it has been known that some environmental chemicals are associated with an increased incidence of cancer in humans. The danger posed by exposure to established human carcinogens such as β-naphthylamine and vinyl chloride was originally recognized from epidemiological evidence. The main purpose of investigating chemical carcinogenesis, however, is to prevent environmentally induced cancer by identifying such chemicals before they are released into the environment. Over the past two or three decades, carcinogenic activity has usually been determined by the ability of a chemical to produce tumours in laboratory animals during lifetime exposure to the chemical. Long-term animal studies of this kind may last for two or three years and utilize scarce resources and expertise. In consequence, it is only feasible to test a very small proportion of the new chemicals produced each year in animal bioassays.

Many attempts were made in the late 1960s and early 1970s to detect potentially carcinogenic chemicals in tests using bacteria or cultured mammalian cells. It was suspected that many cancers resulted from changes to the informational macromolecules of cells, i.e. deoxyribonucleic acid (DNA), and, in general, the tests were based on the induction of genetic changes to the test cells such as gene mutations and chromosomal aberrations. Little progress was made until it was realized that the majority of carcinogenic chemicals required biotransformation by mammalian enzymes before they were in a molecular form capable of interaction with DNA. This observation led to the development, by Professor Bruce Ames and his colleagues at the University of California, USA, of a bacterial test for mutagens that incorporated essential aspects of mammalian metabolism in the form of an enzyme-rich fraction of mammalian liver. In this system, known as the "salmonella assay" or the "Ames test", it was shown that a number of chemicals, known to be carcinogenic in laboratory animal studies, were metabolized by the incorporated mammalian enzymes to reactive molecules that induced mutations in the Salmonella typhimurium tester strains. In a series of validation studies with the salmonella assay conducted during the mid-1970s and totalling about 500 chemicals, a high percentage of carcinogenic chemicals induced mutations in the bacteria and a high proportion of non-carcinogens were negative.

Considering that the salmonella assay could produce results within a week (compared with the two or three years for a rodent bioassay), it is not surprising that it was soon being used extensively throughout the world. Many hundreds of chemicals of diverse structure were tested and, in many cases, interpreted in human health terms without full comprehension of the biological principles involved in extrapolating data from a simple bacterial assay to a complex organism like man. It became apparent at this time that a number of established animal carcinogens consistently gave negative results in the salmonella assay and, similarly, some chemicals, considered to be non-carcinogenic, were shown to be mutagenic in bacterial tests. This observation confirmed that no single short-term assay could be relied on to detect all carcinogens and also confirmed the value of the practice of using short-term *in vitro* and *in vivo* tests in batteries or in tier systems. The variety of such packages proliferated, leading to a great deal of confusion and conflict regarding the most appropriate tests to investigate chemicals for possible carcinogenic activity.

Concern about the reliability, sensitivity and the choice of short-term tests resulted in the instigation of the International Collaborative Programme for the Evaluation of Short-Term Tests for Carcinogens (IPESTTC). This project, completed in 1981, involved investigators from more than 50 laboratories, and some 30 *in vitro* and *in vivo* assays were evaluated for their ability to discriminate between carcinogenic and non-carcinogenic chemicals (de Serres and Ashby, 1981). Twenty-five known carcinogens and 17 chemicals considered to be non-carcinogenic, including 14 pairs of carcinogen/non-carcinogen analogues, were tested in most of the assays. An evaluation of the data indicated that the salmonella mutation assay gave the best overall performance, producing reliable results in a large number of laboratories. Other assays that also appeared to discriminate between carcinogens and non-carcinogens included *in vitro* tests for chromosomal aberrations and

Introduction

unscheduled DNA synthesis and, although fewer chemicals were tested, results from drosophila tests, mammalian cell gene mutation assays, and rodent bone marrow cytogenetic studies suggested that they, too, were useful components of a testing battery. Following a critical evaluation of the data from the IPESTTC project, it was concluded that, although the value of the salmonella assay was confirmed, there were still some rodent carcinogens that were either reproducibly negative in this assay or detected only with difficulty. A proportion of these chemicals were detected in some of the other assays but the data base was insufficient to identify which *in vitro* or *in vivo* test(s) were the most effective complementary assay(s) to the salmonella test.

It was apparent from the IPESTTC study that a further collaborative exercise would be necessary to establish a) the most effective combination of *in vitro* assays for primary screening of chemicals for carcinogenic potential and b) the most useful short-term *in vivo* procedures for confirming mammalian genotoxicity and carcinogenic potential. A collaborative programme designed to investigate these two questions was proposed by the International Programme on Chemical Safety (IPCS) and the National Institute of Environmental Health Sciences (NIEHS) of the USA. Because of the logistical problems involved in organizing and managing international collaborative projects, this programme was divided into two discrete studies. The first, referred to as the Collaborative Study on Short-Term Tests for Genotoxicity and Carcinogenicity (CSSTT/1) was published in 1985 (Ashby et al., 1985) and summarized in Environmental Health Criteria 47 (WHO, 1985). The second part of the programme was the Collaborative Study on Short-Term *In Vivo* Tests for Mutagens and Carcinogens (CSSTT/2) and is the subject of this report.

It was decided very early in the planning stage that, whereas 42 chemicals were investigated in the IPESTTC project, the CSSTT/1 study would concentrate on generating a more comprehensive data base on a smaller number of chemicals rather than an incomplete set of data from a large number. Thus, ten organic chemicals were selected comprising eight established carcinogens that were either negative or difficult to detect in the salmonella assay and two chemicals that had not shown any evidence of carcinogenicity in rodent cancer bioassays. The results of the study were evaluated at a meeting of investigators in 1983 at which data from nearly 90 individual sets of assays conducted by some 60 participating scientists were scrutinised. Almost all the *in vitro* assays in use at that time were represented and four assays, in particular, performed well enough to be considered as possible complementary tests to the salmonella assay. These were tests for chromosomal aberrations, gene mutations and neoplastic transformation in cultured mammalian cells, and an assay for aneuploidy induction in yeast. An important component of the project was to identify protocol variations that might explain differences in results between investigators using, ostensibly, the same assay. This assessment indicated that the protocols in general use for gene mutation and transformation assays in mammalian cells and aneuploidy in yeast require further evaluation before they can be considered fully reproducible between laboratories. The data provided by the investigators using chromosomal aberration assays allowed the working group to identify certain critical factors in the protocols that appeared to influence sensitivity and selectivity in response to carcinogens. The *in vitro* test for chromosomal aberrations was, therefore, considered to be the most appropriate complementary assay to the salmonella test and it was concluded that a combination of these two assays may provide an efficient primary screen for possible new carcinogens and mammalian mutagens.

2. THE COLLABORATIVE STUDY ON SHORT-TERM *IN VIVO* TESTS FOR MUTAGENS AND CARCINOGENS (CSSTT/2) 1983-1985

In general terms, the *in vitro* part of the collaborative study (CSSTT/1) achieved its targets by indicating a small group of assays that show promise as complementary tests to the salmonella mutation assay. Detailed scrutiny of the data also identified critical aspects of the protocols of these assays that required modification in order to reach the levels of reproducibility, sensitivity, and selectivity already achieved by the salmonella assay. Even so, the IPESTTC study had shown that 7 of 14 presumed non-carcinogens elicited positive responses in many of the *in vitro* assays. In the same study, these seven non-carcinogens were predominantly inactive in a series of short-term *in vivo* tests. The *in vivo* test data presented in the IPESTTC study were limited, i.e. only five investigators provided results from mammalian *in vivo* tests and only a proportion of the chemicals were tested by each investigator. The results suggested that, although some non-carcinogens were positive *in vitro*, they were inactive in *in vivo* short-term tests. The non-carcinogens in two of the carcinogen/non-carcinogen pairs, i.e. benzo[a]pyrene/pyrene (BP/PYR) and 2-acetylaminofluorene/4-acetylaminofluorene (2AAF/4AAF), provided good examples of these different responses.

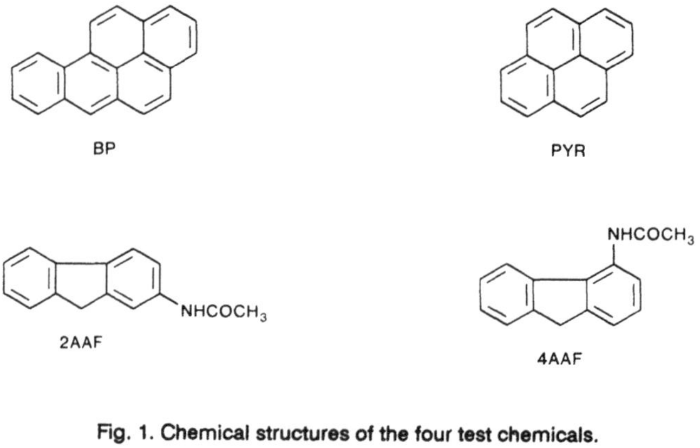

Fig. 1. Chemical structures of the four test chemicals.

These observations were the origin of the present study, the object of which was to generate a comprehensive data profile from a broad range of short-term *in vivo* assays as a means of understanding how various genetic end-points in key target tissues respond to chemicals defined as genotoxic *in vitro*. The objectives and design of the collaborative study on short-term *in vivo* tests (CSSTT/2) were outlined by an *ad hoc* Working Group[a] at a meeting organized by the IPCS in Geneva on 30 April 1981, and the plans were consolidated by an IPCS Working Group[b] in Geneva, on 13-14 November 1981. The subsequent coordination of the collaborative study was the responsibility of a Steering Committee[c] derived primarily from the Working Group.

The four test chemicals selected for the *in vivo* project were the two carcinogen/non-carcinogen pairs, i.e. BP/PYR and 2AAF/4AAF, that provided the initial impetus to the study, and the first samples were distributed to investigators in March 1983. During 1983, additional participants joined the study to provide data on new *in vivo* assays and nine coordinators[d] were appointed to oversee the work being conducted by investigators performing identical or similar assays. In all, 97 investigators from 16 countries participated in CSSTT/2. Progress was reviewed at a meeting of the Steering Group with the coordinators held in Brussels on 12-13 January 1984. At this meeting a plan was developed to enter the data from the study into a computer at NIEHS. It was envisaged that

---

[a] Participants: Dr J. Ashby, Professor N.P. Bochkov, Dr B.E. Matter, Professor T. Matsushima, Dr F.J. de Serres, Dr M. Shelby, and Professor F.H. Sobels.

[b] Participants: Dr J. Ashby, Dr G.R. Douglas, Dr M. Ishidate, Jr., Dr A. Leonard, Dr N. Loprieno, Dr B.E. Matter, Professor T. Matsushima, Dr R. Montesano, Dr F.J. de Serres, Dr M. Shelby, Professor F.H. Sobels, Dr M. Stoltz, and Dr M. Waters.

[c] Steering Committee: Dr F.J. de Serres (Chairman), Dr J. Ashby, Dr. M. Ishidate, Jr., Dr B. Margolin, Dr M. Shelby, Dr M. Draper, and Dr G.C. Becking.

[d] Coordinators: Dr W. Vogel, Dr W.M. Generoso, Dr I.-D. Adler, Dr D. Wild, Dr. T. Tice, Dr B.E. Butterworth, Dr D. McGregor, Dr M. Salamone, and Dr R. Fahrig.

such a plan would allow a comprehensive statistical analysis using common statistical techniques for each kind of assay and provide a comparison of results from different laboratories performing the same assay. Initially, it was expected that all the studies would be completed by October 1984, but by September 1984 it was evident that additional time would be required for many of the investigators to complete their evaluation of the four chemicals. At a second meeting of the Steering Group and coordinators, held on 14-17 November 1984, status reports prepared by the coordinators were reviewed in detail and deadlines were set for the provision of final reports from each investigator. Two additional coordinators were appointed at this meeting to oversee the rodent dominant lethal assay (Dr W. Generoso) and the mouse coat colour spot test (Dr R. Fahrig). Following this progress review, a meet-ing of investigators was planned for May 1985, for the presentation, collation, and assessment of the results and the preparation of final reports on the study.

The meeting of investigators was held during 15-21 May 1985 at Cap d'Agde, France. Representatives from each participating laboratory met to prepare a series of reports comprising a) an assessment of each group of assays, b) summary reports on the germ cell assays and the liver-specific assays, and c) summary reports on the total data base on each pair of chemicals, i.e. BP/PYR and 2AAF/4AAF. During the meeting, draft reports were prepared and were to be finalized during the following two months. At a meeting of the Editors[a] held at NIEHS from 24 July to 6 August 1985, the work group and investigators' reports were reviewed, and a time-table was developed for the completion of all reports and for the preparation of the Introduction and Overview of the study in readiness for final publication of the *in vivo* study.

A feature of both the CSSTT studies and the earlier IPESTTC project was the voluntary participation of a large number of scientists together with support from their

---

[a] Editors: Dr J. Ashby, Dr F.J. de Serres, Dr M.D. Shelby, Dr B.H. Margolin, Dr M. Ishidate, Jr., and Dr G.C. Becking.

parent institutions. The organization of CSSTT/1 and CSSTT/2 was financed largely by IPCS and some of its participating institutions. In most cases, funding of the experimental work was by individual investigators, many of whom incorporated the studies into their research programmes. This, of course, required the goodwill and support of senior management of the participating laboratories from universities, research institutions, and industrial research facilities throughout the world. Additional financial assistance was provided by a number of governments that support IPCS, including Belgium, Italy, Japan, The Netherlands, the United Kingdom, and the USA. The United Kingdom Department of Health and Social Security funded the rat carcinogenicity studies with 2AAF and 4AAF. The Belgian government and its National Institute of Hygiene and Epidemiology financed meetings of the Steering Committee and coordinators in Brussels. The meeting of investigators held in Cap d'Agde was organized by the French government and cosponsored by the French Ministry of Health and the Commission of European Communities.

3. OVERALL AIMS OF THE STUDY AND CRITERIA FOR THE SELECTION OF APPROPRIATE SHORT-TERM *IN VIVO* TESTS

Because of their relative simplicity, reproducibility, and reliability, short-term *in vitro* tests are the methods of choice for the initial testing of chemicals for genotoxic activity. The role and usefulness of genotoxicity assays using whole animals, i.e. short-term *in vivo* tests, are less clearly defined despite the fact that they are widely used and are an integral part of most legislative guidelines for the conduct of mutagenicity tests. In general, *in vivo* tests are more resource-consuming than their *in vitro* counterparts and the use of animals for experiments for which there is an acceptable *in vitro* alternative is to be discouraged. As these observations suggest, *in vivo* assays should be designed to answer questions that cannot be investigated adequately with *in vitro* tests.

3.1 The use of short-term tests for the primary identification of genotoxic chemicals

Certain short-term *in vivo* assays, such as the rodent bone marrow chromosome assay, the rodent dominant lethal test, and the host-mediated assay, were used in the early 1970s in primary screens for the identification of mutagenic chemicals. With the introduction of reliable and valid short-term *in vitro* tests for mutagens in the mid-1970s, the use of *in vivo* procedures for initial screening of chemicals declined considerably. Certain legislative authorities still recommend a combination of *in vitro* tests reserved for confirmatory or supplementary use or for providing data for hazard assessment. These different roles for whole animal procedures have led to the acceptance of test protocols of varying complexity, i.e. less rigorous protocols for screening modes and more comprehensive protocols when the test is required to assess hazard potential.

Implicit in the concept of the two IPCS studies is the assumption that chemicals shown to be genotoxic *in vivo* also exhibit genotoxic activity in a properly designed and conducted *in vitro* primary screen. This principle is well-established in the scientific literature and was confirmed in the IPESTTC and CSSTT/1 studies. Thus, it was an integral principle in the study design that the primary screening of chemicals could be adequately served by *in vitro* tests alone and that short-term *in vivo* assays have no role to play when screening for genotoxic activity. *In vivo* procedures will, therefore, be reserved for more specific applications such as investigating the activity of *in vitro* genotoxins in the whole animal and to assist in the assessment of the mutagenic and carcinogenic potential associated with exposure of humans to *in vitro* genotoxins.

.2 **The use of short-term *in vivo* assays for assessing the hazard associated with exposure to *in vitro* genotoxins**

It is apparent from the last paragraph that the major objective of the study was to investigate the activity in the whole mammal of chemicals identified as genotoxic *in vitro* and to establish which *in vivo* tests are the most useful for this purpose. The major criterion for an acceptable short-term *in vivo* test, therefore, rests with its ability to differentiate between carcinogenic and non-carcinogenic chemicals, particularly those that have been identified as genotoxic in an *in vitro* primary screen. To extend this criterion further, an acceptable assay should be capable of separating carcinogen/non-carcinogen analogues, e.g., 2AAF/4AAF, in which, in some cases, small differences in chemical structure are responsible for dramatic differences in carcinogenic potential. Other important criteria, some of which were more clearly characterized during the course of the study, include the following:

- data should be reproducible between different laboratories,
- the assays should not require too high a degree of technical and scientific expertise to be conducted on a routine, every-day basis,
- the genotoxic changes or end-points of the assays should be clear and unambiguous,
- there should be agreed, valid statistical techniques to differentiate between positive and negative data.

Overall Aims of the Study

It is relevant to the performance of *in vivo* tests to consider the metabolic fate of carcinogenic chemicals. As a generalization and depending on the route of exposure of the animal to the chemicals, reactive metabolites of many carcinogens are generated mainly in the liver as a by-product of a predominantly detoxifying process. These metabolites may be capable of interaction with the genetic material, DNA, in the liver cells, they may be transported in an active form to other tissues, or they may be further modified in those tissues to forms able to interact with DNA. Thus, a study of the genotoxic activity of a chemical in the whole animal should be able to detect the genotoxic effects of chemicals or their metabolites in tissues outside the liver and of those whose main genotoxic reactivity may be confined to the liver itself. For example, assays based on genetic alterations to cells in the bone marrow, which is readily accessible to chemicals or their metabolites circulating in the blood, respond to a wide range of chemical carcinogens. However, where reactive metabolites are not readily transported from the liver, bone marrow-type tests would be of little value and assays capable of detecting the genotoxicity in liver cells should be available.

3.3 The role of short-term *in vivo* tests in research into the mechanisms of cancer

Chemical carcinogenesis is generally recognized as a multistage process that begins with initiation, usually considered to involve changes in DNA structure leading to mutations, followed by promotion of the lesion to a pre-malignant state and progression to overt cancer. Thus, the majority of current short-term tests, designed to detect the consequences of DNA interaction, will only respond to chemicals that may induce tumours by a predominantly genotoxic mechanism or induce the initial phase of the carcinogenic process.

A feature of the literature on short-term tests for chemical carcinogens is the occasional reference to chemicals, shown to be associated with the induction of tumours in laboratory animals, that consistently fail to be detected in short-term *in vitro* or *in vivo* assays for genotoxicity. Such negative observations with established carcinogens have been explained by a lack of sensitivity of the particular assays. If these chemicals (diethylhexylphthalate is an example) are truly non-DNA-reactive, however, then negative data in assays for genotoxicity would be the expected result. The acceptance of the existence of so-called "non-genotoxic carcinogens" is of critical importance to the future of short-term testing and one consideration during the assessment of the CSSTT/2 study was the identification of *in vivo* procedures that may be useful for investigating such chemicals with the eventual objective of developing specific short-term tests for non-DNA-reactive carcinogens.

4 Assays for the detection of germ cell mutagens

As a general principle of genetic toxicology, genetic damage induced by chemicals in somatic cells results in hazard only to the affected individual, while genetic effects in male or female germ cells may cause heritable disease or malformation in the immediate progeny or in future descendants of the affected individual. The majority of the assays represented in the CSSTT/2 study were conducted in cells from somatic tissues and are, therefore, only directly interpretable in terms of somatic mutation and carcinogenic potential. Although there have been attempts to extrapolate data derived from somatic cell assays to assessment of the probability of a chemical inducing germ cell mutations, there are a number of assays, some of which were represented in this study, that measure genetic damage directly in the germ cells. The objectives behind the inclusion of germ cell assays in the present study were to determine:

- which kind of germ cell procedure effectively identifies germ cell mutagens;
- what is the relationship between the induction of changes in sperm morphology and unscheduled DNA synthesis in germ cells and the formation of true heritable mutations;
- which of the four *in vitro* genotoxins induce genetic damage in mammalian germ cells.

4. CRITERIA FOR THE SELECTION OF THE FOUR TEST CHEMICALS

Selection of the two pairs of chemicals, benzo[*a*]pyrene/pyrene (BP/PYR) and 2-acetylaminofluorene/4-acetylaminofluorene (2AAF/4AAF), was based, primarily, on their performance in the IPESTTC study. In that study, seven of the fourteen chemicals believed to be non-carcinogens exhibited a high frequency of positive responses in *in vitro* tests while being predominantly or totally negative in a series of short-term *in vivo* tests. Although the *in vivo* data base was limited, the non-carcinogens in the BP/PYR and 2AAF/4AAF pairs provided good examples of such differences in response and these four chemicals were selected as useful representative candidates for investigating the *in vivo* behaviour of chemicals known to be *in vitro* genotoxins.

4.1 Activity of the four test chemicals in short-term *in vitro* tests

The majority of chemical carcinogens, including BP and 2AAF, require some form of enzyme-mediated biotransformation for the formation of reactive metabolites. Most target cells, whether bacteria, yeast or cultured mammalian cells, used in *in vitro* tests lack the appropriate enzyme activity and this is usually provided in the form of an enzyme-rich fraction derived from homogenates of rat liver, referred to as the S9 fraction. Liver enzyme activity is usually stimulated by pre-treatment of the animals with an enzyme-inducer such as Aroclor 1254.

Both the carcinogens, BP and 2AAF, are consistently positive in bacterial assays and other *in vitro* short-term tests and, with the exception of certain mammalian cell assays, demonstration of genotoxic activity requires the incorporation of a rodent liver enzyme system. Positive results have also be reported for the two non-carcinogens, PYR and 4AAF, in a number of *in vitro* systems but not on the scale nor usually with the same potency as their carcinogenic analogues. Thus, both PYR and 4AAF induce mutations in bacteria, gene conversion in yeast, and unscheduled DNA synthesis (UDS) and gene mutation in cultured mammalian cells. They do not, apparently, induce mutations in yeast or chromosome aberrations in cultured mammalian cells. 4AAF, but not PYR, can induce UDS in cultured primary hepatocytes.

In the salmonella mutation assay, separation of the carcinogen/non-carcinogen pairs is influenced significantly by the nature of the rodent liver activation system employed in the test. When the liver enzyme suspension is derived from uninduced rodents, BP and 2AAF give positive results and the two non-carcinogens, PYR and 4AAF, are generally negative. If Aroclor-induced animals are used as a source of the activation system, however, the ability of the assay to discriminate between the carcinogens and non-carcinogens is lost.

A comprehensive tabulation of the activities of the four chemicals in short-term *in vitro* tests is provided by McGregor (1988b).

2 Summary of carcinogenicity data on the test chemicals

The rodent carcinogenicity data for the four test chemicals is reviewed in Hicks et al. (1988).

Both BP and 2AAF are well established and potent carcinogens in rodents. Fewer studies have been conducted with the non-carcinogens, PYR and 4AAF, and their presumed non-carcinogenicity, although derived from limited rodent bioassays, must remain tentative pending more comprehensive testing.

BP is a locally-acting carcinogen in rats and mice, producing skin tumours after dermal application and tumours of the stomach when administered orally. In mouse skin, it has been shown to have both initiating and promoting activity. BP is also a lung carcinogen in mice and induces mammary gland tumours in rats. There is no evidence that BP is hepatocarcinogenic in rats and only a single, unconfirmed report of the induction of hepatomas in mice. On balance, the available evidence suggests that BP does not induce liver tumours in rodents.

PYR has not been tested for carcinogenic activity in any species other than the mouse and even then, only by dermal application. These studies have shown fairly conclusively that PYR is not carcinogenic by this route.

There is some evidence from promotion/initiation studies on mouse skin that it may have weak initiating activity. Because data on systemic carcinogenesis in the mouse and information from other species are lacking, the carcinogenicity of PYR is somewhat equivocal. However, the fact that its analogue, BP, is such a potent skin carcinogen, whereas the data obtained with PYR in fairly comprehensive mouse skin studies are negative, suggests that the presumed non-carcinogenic status of PYR is justified.

2AAF is a potent carcinogen in both rats and mice. It produces tumours in the liver and bladder in both species after oral administration and in the rat it is carcinogenic in Zymbal's glands and mammary glands. Little information is available about its activity when administered by other routes.

4AAF has only been tested in rats by incorporation in the diet, and its activity in mice has not been investigated. In rat feeding experiments, 4AAF has been consistently non-carcinogenic though there are limited data to suggest that its metabolite, N-OH-4AAF, may have some weak carcinogenic activity. If 4AAF does prove to be carcinogenic, its activity is clearly far less potent than that of 2AAF and further long-term studies are required before 4AAF can be unequivocally regarded as non-carginogenic. The question may be resolved when the results of the rat carcinogenicity study, initiated as part of the CSSTT/2 project, are made available.

5. SOURCE AND PURITY OF THE TEST CHEMICALS

Samples of the four test chemicals were obtained from commercial sources: BP, 2AAF, and 4AAF were supplied by Lancaster Synthesis Ltd., Eastgate, Whiteland, Morecambe, Lancashire, United Kingdom, and PYR was obtained from Aldrich Chemicals, Gillingham, Dorset, United Kingdom. 4AAF was synthesized by a route that avoided contamination with 2AAF. The purity of the chemicals was determined by the supplying laboratories before dispatch to the participants. All the chemicals were greater than 99.5% pure and full analytical details are provided by Paton and Ashby (1988).

6. SHORT-TERM *IN VIVO* ASSAYS

For convenience the assays are divided into six groups:

- cytogenetic (chromosome) assays conducted on cells from rodent bone marrow or other non-hepatic tissues;
- assays investigating a variety of effects in cells from rodent liver;
- miscellaneous assays that utilize other tissues or body fluids;
- mouse coat colour spot tests;
- assays in mammalian germ cells;
- tests utilizing the fruit fly, *Drosophila melanogaster*.

6.1 Cytogenetic assays

Assays for the induction of chromosome aberrations, i.e., microscopically visible alterations in chromosome structure, were conducted in bone marrow cells from rats, mice, and Chinese hamsters and also in mouse ascites tumour cells.

Micronucleus tests were conducted on cells from rat and mouse bone marrow and on erythrocytes in circulating blood from mice. Micronuclei are chromosome fragments or intact chromosomes excluded from the cell nucleus during mitosis. They are considered to be evidence of induced chromosome breakage or chromosome loss and are usually analysed in developing or mature erythrocytes.

Sister chromatid exchanges (SCE) can be demonstrated in metaphase chromosomes by a differential staining technique and occur as a consequence of the exchange of replicating DNA between chromatids at apparently homologous loci. Although considered to result from DNA breakage and reunion, the mechanism of the formation of SCE is not fully understood. Assays for the induction of SCE were conducted in bone marrow cells from rats, mice, and Chinese hamsters, in circulating blood leucocytes from mice, and in Chinese hamster intestinal epithelium.

Table 1. Assays employed in the CSSTT/2 study

1. Cytogenetic studies

   Chromosome aberrations
       Mouse bone marrow
       Mouse ascites tumour cells
       Rat bone marrow
       Chinese hamster bone marrow
   Micronucleus tests
       Mouse bone marrow
       Mouse circulation blood cells
       Rat bone marrow
   Sister chromatid exchanges
       Mouse bone marrow
       Mouse circulating blood lymphocytes
       Rat bone marrow
       Chinese hamster bone marrow
       Chinese hamster intestinal epithelial cells

2. Liver-specific assays

   Tests for initiation/promotion: altered enzyme foci
   Unscheduled DNA synthesis (UDS)
       UDS in mouse liver
       UDS in neonatal, weanling and adult rat liver
   Frequency of S-phase hepatocytes
       S-phase in mouse liver
       S-phase in weanling and adult rat liver
   Cytogenetic tests
       Aberrations in rat liver epithelial-like cells
       SCE in rat liver epithelial-like cells
       Micronuclei in hepatocytes
       Diploid/tetraploid ratio in rat and mouse hepatocytes
   Primary changes in DNA
       Alkaline elution assay for DNA strand damage
       DNA/protein cross-links
       DNA unwinding assay for strand damage

3. Miscellaneous assays

   Specific carcinogenicity assays
       Two-year oral dosing study in rats
       Mouse lung adenoma assay
       Quail egg tumour-induction
   UDS in rat fore-stomach
   Sebaceous gland suppression assay
   Observation of dermal epithelial hyperplasia
   Transformation of rat peritoneal macrophages
   6-Thioguanine-resistant mutations in Syrian hamster lung cells
   Measurement of DNA adducts
       ^{32}P-post-labelling in rat and mouse tissues
       Immunochemical detection of DNA adducts
       Radiolabelled test chemicals - rat liver
   Immunotoxicity assays
       Natural Killer (NK) cell and T-cell cytotoxicity in rats

Table 1 (contd).

3. Miscellaneous assays (contd)

    Host-mediated assays
        Mutation of salmonella in mouse tissues
        Genetic changes in yeast cells in mouse tissues
    Urine mutagenicity tests in rats, mice and guinea pigs

4. Mouse spot tests

    Mouse coat colour spot test
    Mouse melanocyte assay

5. Mammalian germ cell studies

    Dominant lethal assays with male and female mice and male rats
    Morphological abnormalities in mouse and rat spermatozoa
    Unscheduled DNA synthesis in rat and mouse male germ cells

6. Drosophila assays

    Sex-linked recessive lethal mutations in germ cells
    Chromosome loss in germ cells
    Somatic mutation and recombination: mosaic spots in eyes and wings

6.2 Assays in rodent liver cells

A variety of liver-specific assays were represented in the study, including the demonstration of enzyme changes, a number of different tests on DNA, and cytogenetic assays.

The rat liver assay for altered enzyme foci employs a histochemical technique that identifies groups of cells or foci that have elevated levels of the marker enzyme *gamma-*glutamyltranspeptidase (GGT). The observation of GGT-positive foci often precedes the appearance of liver carcinoma and the test is used to attempt to identify early stages of carcinogenesis in the liver. Protocols have been devised to investigate both initiation and promotion stages of carcinogenesis.

A number of investigators used assays that measure directly or indirectly the response of DNA to chemical damage. These included tests for breaks in single strands of DNA using the alkaline elution technique, an assay for the induction of crosslinks between DNA and protein molecules, and a measure of single strand breaks based on the degree of unwinding of DNA molecules. One consequence of

DNA breakage is the initiation of the enzyme-mediated repair process which involves the synthesis of new, relatively short strands of DNA to repair the break. This type of repair is referred to as unscheduled DNA synthesis or UDS (to differentiate from the normal or S-phase DNA synthesis that occurs during cell replication). DNA synthesis can be measured by observing the uptake of tritiated thymidine by the newly synthesized strands using autoradiographical techniques. Assays for the induction of UDS and to measure changes in the numbers of S-phase cells in rodent liver were included in the study.

The cytogenetic methods included the analysis of metaphase chromosome aberrations, micronuclei and SCE in rat liver cells, and the determination of the ratio of diploid to tetraploid cells in rat and mouse liver.

.3 **Miscellaneous assays**

The first group of assays to be considered under this heading are those that are directly related to the induction of tumours in rodents. The most important of these is a 2-year oral dosing study in rats to compare the carcinogenicity of 2AAF and 4AAF. Although the study was not completed at the time of this report, preliminary information from a small group of rats examined after 26 weeks of dosing is available. Also included in this group was a) the mouse lung tumour assay that determined the effects of each of the four test chemicals on the incidence of lung adenoma in mice and b) a test in Japanese quail in which the test chemicals were introduced into the yolk sacs of quail eggs. The birds were then examined for evidence of tumours at various intervals after hatching.

The sebaceous gland suppression test is based on the observation of morphological changes to the sebaceous glands in histological preparations of mouse skin after dermal exposure to the test chemicals. The presence of epidermal hyperplasia can also be detected histologically and both methods have been shown to respond to skin carcinogens, particularly polycyclic hydrocarbons.

Genotoxic carcinogens can bind covalently to biological macromolecules such as DNA either before or after metabolic biotransformation. The products of DNA-binding are referred to as DNA adducts and a number of investigators provided data on the detection and measurement of DNA adducts with the test chemicals in tissues from rats and mice. Three different methods were represented:

- the enzyme-linked immunoabsorbent assay (ELISA);
- the ^{32}P-post-labelling assay;
- an assay for radiolabelled chemicals bound to DNA.

Two similar assays for the investigation of the immune response of animals to exposure to carcinogens were represented. Natural Killer (NK) cells are leucocytes with the ability to lyse a variety of 'foreign' cells, e.g., those with a malignant phenotype. The NK cell assay was used to investigate the capacity of NK cells, derived from the splenic mononuclear leucocytes of rats treated with 2AAF or 4AAF, to lyse human erythroleukaemic cells *in vitro*. The basis of the T-cell assay is that immunocompetent T-cells are able to react to tissue changes induced by carcinogenic chemicals in rats. The changes in T-cell activity can be determined by their cytotoxicity towards target cells derived from rat intestinal adenocarcinoma.

The rat peritoneal cell transformation test is based on the observation that mitogen-stimulated peritoneal cells, harvested from rats dosed with carcinogens, undergo a form of transformation that enables them to proliferate and produce colonies in soft agar culture.

Host-mediated assays were used fairly widely in the early 1970s as primary screening tests for mutagenic chemicals. In its original form, a suspension of microbial target cells, i.e. yeast or bacteria, was introduced into the peritoneal cavities of mice. The mice were treated with the suspect chemical and, after an appropriate interval, the target cells were harvested and changes in the mutation frequency or other genetic end-points were determined in *in vitro* culture. Since that time, there have been several modifications to the procedure, the most significant being the injection of the target organisms into the circulating blood of the host. In this way, the bacterial or yeast target cells are distributed in various organs and can, for example, be harvested from the liver, lungs, and kidney. The target cells can, in principle, be affected by reactive metabolites generated from the test chemical in these organs. Intra-sanguinous host-mediated assays using either Salmonella typhimurium or the yeast, *Saccharomyces cerevisiae*, were represented in the study.

Urine and other body fluids can be collected from rodents treated with test chemicals and assayed for mutagenic activity. For example, after appropriate treatment to release conjugated metabolites, urine can be tested for the presence of mutagens in a conventional *in vitro* bacterial mutation assay. In principle, the urine assay is capable of detecting mutagenic chemicals excreted unchanged or after metabolic activation.

4 The mouse spot test

The mouse spot test detects mutations induced in melanocyte precurser cells in the embryos of specially derived strains of mice. The mouse strain carries recessive mutations at a number of specific coat colour loci and the embryos are, thus, heterozygous at these loci. Mutations induced at the wild-type or normal alleles of the coat colour loci result in the development of clones of the mutant melanocytes. The young mice are examined after birth and the mutations are expressed as patches of contrasting coloured fur. The mutations can result from one of a number of genetic events including gene mutations, chromosome deletions, mitotic crossing-over, and loss of whole chromosomes. In addition to the conventional technique of observing the appearance of coloured spots in the fur, a modification of the spot test allows the microscopic recognition of mutant melanocytes in preparations of embryonic skin.

5 Mammalian germ cell studies

The classical dominant lethal assay in male rodents involves the treatment of the animals with the test chemical and then mating with groups of females at intervals to cover the complete spermatogenic cycle. Dominant lethal mutations induced at any stage of spermatogenesis can be detected by dissection of the uterine contents of each female and are characterized by dead fetuses or a reduction in the numbers of fetal implantations. Dominant lethal assays included in the study were those involving treatment of male rats, male mice, or female mice.

Two other assays represented in this group were the abnormal sperm morphology assay and the unscheduled DNA synthesis (UDS) test. The former assay monitors mature spermatazoa for irregularities in morphology at intervals after treatment of rodents with the test chemicals. The UDS test measures DNA repair in developing spermatocytes and spermatids.

6.6 Drosophila assays

Although data from drosophila tests cannot be regarded as appropriate alternatives to mammalian data for assessing the potential hazard to humans from exposure to genotoxic chemicals, drosophila are, in fact, intact, complex, eukaryotic organisms whose metabolic and genetic characteristics have some parallels with those of the whole mammal. Their main value in genotoxicity testing lies with the availability of assays to study the effects of chemicals on both somatic and germ cells. The tests represented in the CSSTT/2 study were:

- the sex-linked recessive lethal mutation assay in germ cells;
- tests for chromosome loss from germ cells;
- assays for somatic mutation and recombination using the induction of mosaic spots in either the wings or the eyes.

7. RESULTS

The investigators met at Cap d'Agde, France, from 15 to 21 May 1985, to assess the results of the study. Each group of investigators presenting data from a particular type of assay discussed their data and individual results were assessed and agreed. This led to the preparation of consensus reports on the response of each assay to the four test chemicals. These consensus views were then incorporated into coordinators' summary reports on each group of assays. Summary reports were presented and critically discussed in open plenary discussions, thereby allowing the overall conclusions and recommendations resulting from the study to be formulated. Reports of individual investigators, the coordinators summary reports, and certain technical appendices form the main text of the final publication together with an editorial overview of the study (Ashby et al., 1988).

The purpose of this chapter of the report is to present the results of the *in vivo* studies with the four test chemicals and to construct a profile, in qualitative terms, of their genotoxic activity in the whole animal. Quantitative differences in response in relation to sex, species, route of exposure, and technical variations are considered in more detail in the next section, which also includes a comprehensive tabulation of the data generated by individual investigators (Table 4). However, as many of the assays were replicated in a number of laboratories, a simplified table of results is presented here (Table 2). It must be emphasised that Table 2 contains the consensus views of the Working Groups assessing the individual results and performance of each assay and that, in some cases, there were conflicting results on the same assay from participating laboratories.

.1 Benzo[a]pyrene (BP) and pyrene (PYR)

1.1 *Cytogenetic studies*

Assays for the induction of structural chromosome aberrations or micronuclei in rodent bone marrow cells

Results

Table 2. Results of the short-term *in vivo* tests summarized by Working Groups [a]

	BP	PYR	2AAF	4AAF
1. Cytogenetic studies				
Chromosomal aberrations				
Mouse bone marrow	●	●	?	●
Mouse ascites cells	●	NT	●	●
Rat bone marrow	●	●	?	●
Chinese hamster bone marrow	●	●	●	●
Micronucleus tests				
Mouse bone marrow	●	●	●	●
Mouse blood - maternal	●	●	●	●
Mouse blood - fetal	●	●	?	●
Rat bone marrow	●	●	●	●
Sister chromatid exchange				
Mouse bone marrow	●	○	●	○
Mouse blood	●	●	●	●
Rat bone marrow	●	○	●	○
Chinese hamster bone marrow	●	●	●	●
Chinese hamster intestinal cells	●	●	●	●
2. Liver-specific assays				
Altered enzyme foci - rat	●	●	●	○
Unscheduled DNA synthesis				
Mouse liver	●	●	●	●
Rat liver	●	●	●	○
S-phase hepatocytes				
Mouse liver	NT	NT	○	●
Rat liver - adult	○	●	?	●
Rat liver - weanling	●	NT	NT	NT
Cytogenetic tests				
Metaphase aberrations - rat	○	●	○	●
Micronuclei - rat	●	●	●	●
SCE - rat	○	●	?	●
Ploidy - rat	●	●	●	●
Ploidy - mouse	●	●	●	●
Primary DNA changes				
Alkaline elution	●	●	?	?
DNA/protein cross-links	●	●	●	NT
DNA unwinding	●	●	●	●
with repair inhibitor	●	●	●	●
3. Miscellaneous assays				
Carcinogenicity				
Oral dosing - rat	NT	NT	●	?
Mouse lung adenoma	●	●	●	●
Quail egg tumours	?	?	?	?
UDS in rat fore-stomach	?	●	●	●
Sebacious gland suppression - mouse	●	●	NT	NT
Epithelial hyperplasia - mouse	●	●	NT	NT
Peritoneal macrophages - rat	●	●	●	●
Syrian hamster lung - mutation	●	●	?	●

Evaluation of Short-term Tests for Carcinogens (In Vivo)

Table 2 (contd).

			BP	PYR	2AAF	4AAF
3.	Miscellaneous assays (contd)					
	DNA adducts					
		^{32}P-post-labelling - rat	●	●	●	○
		Immunochemical (ELISA)	NT	NT	?	?
		Radiolabelled chemicals	NT	NT	●	●
	Immunotoxicity					
		Natural Killer (NK) cells	NT	NT	●	●
		T-cell cytoxicity	●	●	●	○
	Host-mediated assays - mouse					
		Salmonella typhimurium	●	●	●	●
		Saccharomyces (liver)	●	●	●	●
		Saccharomyces (lung)	●	●	●	●
	Urine mutagenicity					
		Rats	●	●	●	●
		Mice	○	○	●	●
		Guinea-pig	NT	NT	●	NT
4.	Mouse spot tests					
		Coat colour spots	●	●	●	●
		Melanocyte assays	NT	NT	●	●
5.	Mammalian germ cells					
	Dominant lethal assays					
		Male mice	●	●	●	●
		Female mice	●	●	●	●
		Male rats	NT	NT	●	●
	Sperm abnormalities					
		Mice	●	●	●	●
		Rats	NT	NT	●	●
	UDS in germ cells					
		Mice	●	●	●	●
		Rats	●	●	●	●
6.	Drosophila assays					
		Sex-linked recessives	●	●	●	●
		Chromosome loss	●	●	●	●
	Somatic mutation					
		Eye spots	●	●	●	●
		Wing spots	●	●	○	?

[a] ● = positive
○ = weak positive
◐ = negative
? = results inconclusive or not yet reported
NT = not tested

Results

were consistently positive with BP and negative with PYR. Among a number of experimental variables between different investigators, neither the species, strain, sex, solvent, nor route of exposure affected the qualitative result. BP increased the incidence of sister chromatid exchanges (SCE) in mouse, rat, and Chinese hamster bone marrow in every study. The results with PYR, however, were less clear, and this presumed non-carcinogen induced SCE at high dose levels in mice after oral or intraperitoneal dosing and in male rats after oral administration, i.e. 3 of 9 SCE studies reported a weak positive result. Analysis of micronuclei in circulating blood erythrocytes from maternal, fetal, or weanling mice, and SCE in circulating blood lymphocytes from adult mice clearly discriminated between BP and PYR.

7.1.2   *Liver-specific assays*

Five investigators provided data from observations of altered enzyme foci in rat liver under the general heading of initiation/promotion assays. There were, however, significant protocol variations between investigators. Two protocols required administration of the rodent tumour promotor, phenobarbitone, in the drinking-water or diet for some weeks after dosing in order to determine initiating activity of the test chemicals. The promoting activity of the test chemicals was studied by two other workers by producing initiation events in the liver before treatment with the test chemicals. The fifth protocol tested the ability of the chemicals to induce both initiation and promotion without discriminating between the two phases. In all cases, the evidence for induced pre-cancerous changes was the observation of foci or clones of cells with altered enzyme characteristics. BP was shown to have significant initiating activity in rat liver in two studies and, in a third study, was shown capable of promoting nitrosamine-induced initiation. Using a fourth, essentially experimental, protocol that involved the transplantation of donor liver cells to the host animal, BP failed to show promoting activity. No evidence of tumour initiating or promoting activity was observed in any of the studies with PYR.

The rodent liver assay for unscheduled DNA synthesis measures the induction of repairable lesion in the DNA of hepatocytes and, theoretically, should be capable of detecting chemicals that are metabolized in the liver to produce genotoxic (i.e. DNA-interactive) metabolites. Both BP and PYR were reproducibly negative in mouse hepatocytes and in hepatocytes from adult, weanling, or neonatal rats using either oral or intraperitoneal dosing. The induction of S-phase DNA synthesis was also investigated and BP was shown to increase the incidence of S-phase cells in weanling rats and, in one of two experiments, a slight increase in S-phase cells was observed in adult rats. In mice, BP had no significant effect on the incidence of S-phase, and PYR showed no evidence of S-phase synthesis induction in either species.

Limited data were presented on the cytogenetic effects of the chemicals in liver-derived cells. In epithelial-like cells from weanling rats, BP was observed to induce a small increase in the incidence of structural chromosome aberrations and SCE; tests with PYR were negative. These findings, however, require confirmation. No evidence of micronucleus-induction was detected in rats treated with BP or PYR after partial hepatectomy. Using a cytofluorometric method, an increase in the ratio of diploid to tetraploid cells was observed in liver-derived cells after treatment of rats with BP, but not after dosing with PYR.

Three different assays were used to study the ability of the chemicals to induce single-strand breaks (SSB) in liver cell DNA. Both BP and PYR were uniformly negative in the alkaline elution assay for SSB conducted in three laboratories. BP, however, was shown to induce crosslinks between DNA and protein, while PYR was negative in this assay. The third assay in this group was a measure of SSB based on the degree of alkali-induced unwinding of DNA molecules. When the DNA-repair inhibitor, adenosine arabinoside was incorporated, BP was shown to induce SSB in mouse liver cell DNA using this technique. In the absence of the repair inhibitor, SSB were not observed. PYR produced negative results in the DNA-unwinding assay. The results from this group of assays suggest that BP is capable of inducing SSB in the DNA of mouse liver cells that are effectively repaired in the absence of a DNA-repair inhibitor. In rats, the observation of DNA/protein crosslinks tentatively suggests the induction of SSB in

Results

rat liver cells, but additional studies are required to assess the DNA effects of BP in rat liver.

7.1.3 *Miscellaneous assays*

Two investigators are producing data that are directly related to the induction of tumours. In the lung adenoma assay, mice were injected with BP or PYR by the intraperitoneal route, 2-3 times each week, for up to 8 weeks. The mice were examined 23 weeks after the start of the study and the numbers of adenoma on the surface of the pulmonary lobes were recorded. BP induced a significant increase in adenomas compared with the untreated control group while no increase in the induction of these tumours was observed in mice injected with PYR. This assay differentiated very clearly between the carcinogenic activity of BP and PYR. The second study in this category involved injecting the test material into the yolk sac of quail eggs and then observing the birds for the presence of tumours at intervals after hatching. In birds examined at approximately 3 months, there was no evidence of tumour induction by either BP or PYR. Surviving birds will be maintained for up to 12 months before being examined for the presence of tumours and, therefore, a definitive conclusion on the carcinogenicity of BP and PYR to quail is not yet possible.

One investigator studied the induction of UDS in the fore-stomach of rats after oral dosing; the data with BP were considered to be equivocal while PYR gave negative results.

Two assays involved the application of the test chemicals to mouse skin followed by histological examination of skin sections. BP induced epithelial hyperplasia and suppression of sebaceous glands, both of which have been correlated with polycyclic hydrocarbon-induced skin carcinogenesis. PYR failed to elicit either of these responses.

The transformation of rat peritoneal macrophages has been advocated as a short-term *in vivo* test for potentially carcinogenic chemicals. Macrophages isolated from rats dosed with BP or PYR, however, failed to show any evidence of transformation in experiments conducted in three laboratories.

Somatic mutation data on cells isolated from Syrian hamster lung tissue, after dosing with the test chemicals, were presented by one investigator. Cultures of cells from animals dosed with BP showed a higher frequency of mutations at the 6-thioguanine locus than those from untreated hamsters, suggesting the induction of somatic mutations in lung cells from this species. PYR produced negative mutation data in this assay.

^{32}P-labelling of purified DNA was used to detect DNA adducts in tissues from rats and mice treated intraperitoneally with the test chemicals. Measurable levels of PYR adducts were not detected in DNA from mouse liver, lung, or kidney, or from rat liver or lung tissues. BP adducts were identified in all of these tissues.

Only one of the two assays for immunotoxicity was conducted with the BP/PYR pair. Thus, the T-cell assay showed that BP, but not PYR, was capable of inducing a cytotoxic response in rat T-cells.

Two investigators provided data from host-mediated assays in mice dosed with BP or PYR. In tests with the yeast, *Saccharomyces cerevisiae*, a significant increase in mitotic gene conversion was detected in yeast cells isolated from the liver of mice dosed with either BP or PYR, while yeast cells isolated from lung tissue produced negative data with both chemicals. No evidence of the induction of mutations was observed in Salmonella typhimurium isolated from liver tissues of mice dosed with BP or PYR.

Assays for the detection of mutagens in urine were conducted with both rats and mice. Mutagenic activity was detected in urine samples from both species after dosing with BP or PYR and, therefore, the test failed to differentiate between the two chemicals.

1.4 *Mouse spot tests*

Only one investigator provided mouse spot test data on BP and PYR. Using the observation of coat colour spots in

Results

off-spring as evidence of somatic mutation, BP was clearly positive and PYR negative.

7.1.5 Mammalian germ cell assays

BP induced dominant lethal mutations in both male and female mice after intraperitoneal injections but not after oral dosing. The response in the male was highly stage-specific; only the mature spermatozoa were sensitive and spermatid and spermatocyte stages were unaffected. Dominant lethal assays with PYR were reproducibly negative.

Studies of morphological abnormalities in mature spermatozoa were conducted in mice after oral or intraperitoneal dosing. BP was uniformly positive in this assay, regardless of the route of exposure. Although a weak positive response was observed in one of seven experiments with PYR, this observation was not confirmed and the consensus view was that PYR did not induce sperm abnormalities. In studies of the induction of unscheduled DNA synthesis in rat and mouse male germ cells, negative results were obtained with both BP and PYR.

7.1.6 Drosophila assays

In all, ten studies were conducted with BP and PYR in drosophila and in each case the oral route of treatment was used. Germ cell studies, i.e. the sex-linked recessive lethal mutation assay and the test for chromosome loss, were uniformly negative with both chemicals. In contrast, tests for somatic mutation and recombination, based on the observation of eye or wing spots, showed that BP was able to induce genetic changes in somatic cells in each of three studies. PYR was consistently negative.

7.2 2-Acetylaminofluorene and 4-acetylaminofluorene

7.2.1 Cytogenetic studies

Seven investigators provided data from analysis of metaphase chromosomes in mouse bone marrow cells. 2AAF induced a significant increase in the incidence of structural chromosome aberrations in only two of seven assays, one of which was considered to be inconclusive.

The results of assays with 4AAF were negative with the exception of two assays in which the data were inconclusive. In contrast, 2AAF was reproducibly positive and 4AAF consistently negative in 15 of 16 micronucleus tests conducted in mouse bone marrow erythrocytes. The route of exposure, i.e. oral dosing or intraperitoneal injection, did not appear to influence the outcome of these studies. Micronuclei were produced by 2AAF in rat bone marrow cells and a small increase was also recorded in one of two assays with 4AAF. Two workers investigated the influence of these two chemicals on the incidence of structural chromosome aberrations in Chinese hamster bone marrow; 2AAF was positive in this species and 4AAF gave a weak positive result in one of the two studies. Both chemicals failed to induce detectable chromosome damage in mouse ascites tumour cells. Four micronucleus tests were conducted with mouse blood erythrocytes. An increase in micronuclei was recorded by one worker in blood cells from weanling mice dosed with 2AAF, although when samples of maternal or fetal blood were examined, increases in micronuclei were not apparent. However, studies conducted in another laboratory showed that 2AAF was capable of increasing the incidence of micronuclei in fetal blood. Thus, 2AAF is clearly clastogenic to rodent bone marrow cells while 4AAF was considered by most investigators to be devoid of clastogenic activity.

Nine assays for sister chromatid exchanges (SCE) were conducted in bone marrow cells from mice, rats, or Chinese hamsters. 2AAF was clearly positive in this test and the consensus view was that 4AAF, although negative in four assays, was capable of inducing a small (but significant) increase in SCE. In studies with mouse lymphocytes and Chinese hamster intestinal epithelial cells, 2AAF was positive and 4AAF was considered to be negative.

2.2 Liver-specific assays

As discussed in section 7.1.2, there were a number of variations between the five protocols used in the initiation/promotion assays. Significant initiation and promotion activity was demonstrated in studies with 2AAF based on the observation of foci of cells with altered enzyme characteristics in rat liver. These assays failed

Results

to discriminate clearly between the two chemicals, since 4AAF was shown to be an initiator in the hands of one investigator and had weak promoting activity in another study. Both chemicals, therefore, proved capable of producing these pre-cancerous changes in rat liver tissue though with different degrees of potency.

2AAF and 4AAF failed to induce detectable unscheduled DNA synthesis (UDS) in mouse hepatocytes after oral dosing. Quite different results were obtained in rat liver, however, and 2AAF was shown to induce UDS in rat hepatocytes in each of the seven laboratories that submitted data. Three of these laboratories also reported the detection of a small increase in UDS in rats after dosing with 4AAF. The other four laboratories obtained negative data. Thus, 2AAF induced UDS in hepatocytes from rats but not mice, and 4AAF elicited a weak UDS response in the rat and was negative in mouse cells.

The results of the analysis of S-phase DNA synthesis indicated that the presumed non-carcinogen, 4AAF, was a very potent inducer of S-phase cells in the liver of both rats and mice. 2AAF, on the other hand, induced only a small increase in S-phase cells in the mouse and three studies in rat liver produced one clear positive and two negative results.

In cytogenetic experiments in cells derived from rat liver, 2AAF appeared to induce a small increase in the incidence of structural aberrations and, in partially hepatectomised rats, a significant increase in micronuclei. 4AAF gave negative results in tests for chromosomal aberrations, micronuclei, and SCE in rat liver cells. When the ratio of diploid to tetraploid cells was investigated in rat and mouse liver, an increase in the ratio was observed in both species after dosing with 2AAF but not in response to 4AAF.

The alkaline elution assay for single strand breaks (SSB) produced conflicting results between three laboratories. Two investigators presented negative data from assays with both chemicals while a third observed that both 2AAF and 4AAF produced SSB in this test. Using the detection of DNA/DNA or DNA/protein crosslinks as a measure of SSB, 2AAF was shown to produce SSB. No data were presented on 4AAF. Another investigator calculated

SSB from the amount of DNA unwinding induced by the chemicals. 2AAF and 4AAF gave positive and negative results, respectively, either in the presence or absence of a DNA repair inhibitor. These data suggest that, unlike 4AAF, 2AAF is capable of producing SSB in rat liver DNA under appropriate experimental conditions.

2.3 Miscellaneous assays

A 2-year oral dosing carcinogenicity study in rats with 2AAF and 4AAF is still in progress. Preliminary findings in a small number of animals examined after 26 weeks of dosing showed that an increase in liver tumours was already apparent in animals dosed with 2AAF; there was no evidence of tumour induction in the 4AAF-dosed animals.

The lung adenoma assay, in which mice were given intraperitoneal injections of the test chemicals 2-3 times a week for up to 8 weeks, clearly separated 2AAF and 4AAF. 2AAF induced a significant increase in adenomas while the incidence in mice dosed with 4AAF was comparable with that of untreated mice.

There was no evidence of the induction of UDS in rat fore-stomach after oral dosing with either chemical, and the assay for the induction of somatic mutations in Syrian hamster lung cells produced inconclusive data with 2AAF and was negative in tests with 4AAF. The rat macrophage test was reproducibly negative with both 2AAF and 4AAF.

Three techniques were applied to detect the presence of DNA adducts formed in various tissues after dosing rodents with the test chemicals. Data from the ELISA technique, which requires the use of monoclonal antibodies to detect specific adducts, are not yet available. However, the ^{32}P-post-labelling method indicated that 2AAF formed adducts with DNA in rat liver and lung and in mouse liver, lung, and kidney after intraperitoneal dosing. No data were presented from mice dosed with 4AAF. In the rat, however, 4AAF formed adducts in liver and lung DNA though at a much lower rate than 2AAF. In studies using radiolabelled test materials, both chemicals were shown to form adducts with DNA in the liver and lungs of rats after

Results

intraperitoneal administration, although adduct formation was considerably less with 4AAF than with 2AAF.

2AAF produced positive results in both immunotoxicity assays. However, although 4AAF was negative in the Natural Killer (NK) cell assay, data from the T-cell cytotoxicity test suggested that it was capable of inducing a measurable cytotoxic response in rat T-Cells.

Nine sets of data were considered from mouse host-mediated assays. In eight of these, including assays for genetic changes in yeast isolated from liver, lung and kidney, and for mutations in salmonella isolated from liver tissue, 4AAF was uniformly negative. 2AAF produced two weak positive responses and five negative results in the same eight studies. The ninth assay, however, indicated that both chemicals induced mitotic gene conversion in yeast isolated from liver tissue. In addition, mutagenic materials were detected in urine samples from rats and mice after dosing with either isomer and from guinea-pigs after dosing with 2AAF. 4AAF data on guinea-pig urine were not available.

7.2.4 Mouse spot tests

Six separate mouse spot tests were conducted with 2AAF and the results were equally divided between positive and negative. An increase in coat colour spots was detected in two studies while in two others, no evidence of the induction of coat colour spots was observed. Similarly, in the melanocyte assay, one positive result and one negative were reported. Four of five spot tests conducted with 4AAF were negative and the data were inconclusive in the fifth.

7.2.5 Mammalian germ cell assays

Dominant lethal mutation assays conducted in male or female mice ΰ male rats and tests for the induction of UDS in rat or mouse male germ cells were uniformly negative with both compounds. In the test for morphological abnormalities in mature spermatozoa, two assays in which 2AAF was given orally to mice or rats were also negative. After intraperitoneal dosing, however, 2AAF induced a significant increase in the incidence of abnormal mouse sperm. 4AAF was negative in both species regardless of the route of exposure. These data suggest that, although 2AAF or its metabolites appear capable of penetrating the testes and adversely affecting sperm morphology after intraperitoneal dosing, there is no evidence for interaction of 2AAF metabolites with germ cell DNA.

2.6 Drosophila assays

The mutagenic effects of the two chemicals on drosophila germ cells were studied in tests for sex-linked recessive lethal mutations in five laboratories and for chromosome loss in two laboratories. Data from six of these studies indicated that neither chemical produced genetic damage in drosophila. In the seventh laboratory, however, 2AAF was clearly mutagenic in the sex-linked recessive lethal assay; 4AAF produced a weak positive result in this study.

2AAF induced eye or wing spots in somatic mutation and recombination assays in drosophila, although the response was weak in two of the studies. The somatic mutation data generated from tests with 4AAF were ambiguous, producing one weak positive result, one inconclusive result and one negative.

3 Summary of the *in vivo* genotoxicity of the four chemicals

A comprehensive *in vivo* genotoxicity profile has been generated on the four test chemicals, each of which had previously shown evidence of mutagenic activity in *in vitro* screening tests. It is relevant, in this section, to consider the mammalian genotoxicity in relation to the hazard assessment procedures recommended by many regulatory bodies. Table 3 shows the mutagenic activity of the chemicals in the *in vivo* tests common to most legislative guidelines. Based on these results, and in the absence of pharmacokinetic and metabolic data, BP would be considered to present a potential mutagenic and carcinogenic hazard and 2AAF would be regarded as a potential carcinogen. These observations are, of course, corroborated by the established carcinogenic activity of these two chemicals.

The abbreviated data base shown in Table 3 suggests that neither 4AAF nor PYR present a significant genotoxic

Results

hazard and it is useful to consider whether the comprehensive data generated in CSSTT/2 support this initial prediction. The summarized consensus results (Table 2) show that conclusive data for PYR were presented from 48 distinct *in vivo* tests and PYR was considered to be negative in 43 of these. The remaining five tests suggested a weak induction of SCE in rodent bone marrow that was not reproduced in all laboratories, a single positive host-mediated assay, and evidence of the excretion of mutagenic metabolites in rodent urine. None of these data seriously question the validity of the original prediction that PYR is not a significant genotoxic hazard.

Table 3. Activity of the four test chemicals in established *in vivo* mutagenicity assays

	BP	PYR	2AAF	4AAF
Somatic cell tests				
Metaphase chromosome analysis	●	○	●[a]	○
Micronucleus test	●	●	●	○
Mouse spot test	●	○	●[a]	○
Germ cell tests				
Dominant lethal assay	●	○	○	○
Heritable translocation test	NT	NT	NT	NT
Mammalian germ cell cytogenetics	NT	NT	NT	NT

[a] Data not consistent between laboratories
NT = not tested
● = positive   ○ = negative

A similar analysis of the 4AAF data indicates that conclusive results were obtained from 50 different types of *in vivo* tests. Of these, 38 were regarded as negative and the remaining twelve assays produced positive or weak positive results. Like BP, 4AAF produced a positive result in a host-mediated assay and in tests for mutagenic activity in rodent urine. Other observations, however, suggest that 4AAF may not be devoid of *in vivo* genotoxicity. For example, 4AAF induced detectable unscheduled DNA synthesis in rat liver hepatocytes that was reproduced in three different laboratories. One investigator reported the induction of micronuclei in rat bone marrow cells after intraperitoneal dosing with 4AAF, and five of seven studies conducted in rat or mouse bone marrow recorded small, but significant, increases in SCE. There was also data to suggest that 4AAF was capable of adduct formation with liver cell DNA in rats. All the germ cell data on 4AAF were negative. The positive findings in somatic tissues cannot be dismissed as inconsequential and they raise serious doubts about the prediction, based on the data shown in Table 3, that 4AAF does not present a significant genotoxic hazard. The outcome of the 2-year rat carcinogenicity study with 4AAF is crucial to the assessment of the validity of this prediction and, in fact, to the evaluation of the whole CSSTT/2 data base.

8. ASSESSMENT OF THE PERFORMANCE OF THE ASSAYS

The purpose of this section is to present an objective assessment of the performance of the *in vivo* tests as it relates to the carcinogenic activity of the test chemicals. (A detailed tabulation of the qualitative results of each assay is presented in Table 4). Data from a study of only four chemicals do not, of course, provide sufficient information on which to judge the overall value of a particular assay for discriminating between non-carcinogenic and potentially carcinogenic chemicals. However, when a data base of this magnitude is available, in which many tests were replicated in a number of different laboratories, then a unique insight into the utility, reproducibility, and reliability, as well as the accuracy of the tests, can be obtained. Thus, data from the current study, together with the considerable experience of the investigators and assessors, enable the performance of many of the assays to be comprehensively evaluated.

Although a high proportion of test systems performed reasonably well with these four chemicals, some assays, not surprisingly, failed to meet the predetermined criteria for acceptable performance (section 4). The rodent host-mediated and urine mutagenicity assays are good examples. They involve either the exposure of marker organisms to the chemicals or its metabolites *in vivo* or the detection of mutagenic excretory products in urine of treated rodents. Both types of tests were conducted in several laboratories and neither proved capable of identifying the two carcinogens among the four *in vitro* mutagens, i.e. the host-mediated assays were generally negative with the four test chemicals while the urine tests were uniformly positive. These observations suggest that neither of these two classes of tests has any practical value in evaluating the *in vivo* genotoxicity of chemicals known to be genotoxic *in vitro*. The results obtained from the peritoneal macrophage transformation assay suggest a similar conclusion. This is a form of host-mediated assay in which the transformation of macrophages, isolated from the peritoneum of treated rats, is investigated in *in vitro* culture. The four test chemicals gave negative results in each of three laboratories.

Evaluation of Short-term Tests for Carcinogens (In Vivo)

Table 4. IPCS CSSTT *in vivo* study –
summary of qualitative results from individual investigators[a]

Assay			Chapter numbers[b]	BP	PYR	2AAF	4AAF	Route of exposure
1.	**CYTOGENETICS**							
1.1.	Chromosomal aberrations							
	1.1.1	Mouse bone marrow	8	●	○	NT	NT	o
			8	NT	NT	●	?	ip
	1.1.2	Mouse bone marrow	9	●	○	NT	NT	o
			9	NT	NT	○	○	ip
	1.1.3	Mouse bone marrow	10	●	○	○	○	o
	1.1.4	Mouse bone marrow	11	●	○	●	○	o
	1.1.5	Mouse bone marrow	12	●	○	○	?	o
	1.1.6	Mouse bone marrow	13	●	NT	○	○	o
	1.1.7	Mouse bone marrow	14	●	○	?	○	ip
	1.1.8	Mouse ascites tumour cells	13	●	NT	○	○	o
	1.1.9	Rat bone marrow	15	●	○	NT	NT	o
			15	NT	NT	?	○	ip
	1.1.10	Chinese hamster bone marrow	16	●	○	●	○	o
	1.1.11	Chinese hamster bone marrow	17	○	○	○	○	o
1.2	Micronuclei							
	1.2.1	Mouse bone marrow	19	●	○	●	○	o
	1.2.2	Mouse bone marrow	20	●	○	●	○	o
	1.2.3	Mouse bone marrow	21	●	○	●	○	o
	1.2.4	Mouse bone marrow	22	●	○	●	○	o
	1.2.5	Mouse bone marrow	23	●	○	●	○	o
	1.2.6	Mouse bone marrow	24	●	○	●	○	o
	1.2.7	Mouse bone marrow	25	●	○	NT	NT	o
	1.2.8	Mouse bone marrow	26	●	○	●	○	o
	1.2.9	Mouse bone marrow	27	●	○	●	○	o
	1.2.10	Mouse bone marrow	28	●	○	NT	NT	o
			28	NT	NT	●	○	ip
	1.2.11	Mouse bone marrow	29	●	○	●	○	ip
	1.2.12	Mouse bone marrow	29	●	○	NT	NT	o
	1.2.13	Mouse bone marrow	30	●	○	●	○	o
			30	●	○	●	○	ip
	1.2.14	Mouse bone marrow	31	●	○	●	○	ip
	1.2.15	Mouse bone marrow	32	●	○	●	○	o
	1.2.16	Mouse bone marrow	33	●	○	●	○	o
	1.2.17	Mouse blood - weanling	34	●	○	●	?	o
	1.2.18	Mouse blood - fetal	34	●	○	●	○	o
	1.2.19	Mouse blood - maternal	34	●	○	●	○	o
	1.2.20	Mouse blood - fetal	32	●	○	●	○	o
	1.2.21	Rat bone marrow	35	NT	NT	●	○	o
	1.2.22	Rat bone marrow	36	●	○	NT	NT	o
			36	NT	NT	●	○	ip
1.3	Sister chromatid exchange							
	1.3.1	Mouse bone marrow	38	●	○	●	○	ip
	1.3.2	Mouse bone marrow	39	●	○	●	○	o

Assessment of the Performance of the Assays

Table 4 (contd).

1.3.3		Mouse bone marrow	40	●	○	●	○	o
1.3.4		Mouse bone marrow	41	●	○	●	○	ip
1.3.5		Mouse bone marrow	42	●	○	●	○	o
1.3.6		Mouse bone marrow	43	●	○	○	○	o
1.3.7		Rat bone marrow	44	●	○	●	○	o
1.3.8		Mouse lymphocytes	45	●	○	●	○	o
1.3.9		Chinese hamster bone marrow	46	●	○	●	○	ip
		Chinese hamster bone marrow	46	●	○	●	○	o
1.3.10		Chinese hamster intestinal cells	46	●	○	●	○	o
2.	**LIVER-SPECIFIC ASSAYS**							
2.1	Initiation/promotion							
2.1.1		Altered enzyme foci	50	NT	NT	○	○	o
2.1.2		GGT-positive foci	51	●	○	●	○	o
2.1.3		GGT-positive foci	52	●	○	●	●	o
2.1.4		GGT-positive foci - promotion	53	●	○	●	○	o
2.1.5		GGT-positive foci	54	○	○	●	○	o
2.1.6		GGT-positive foci	73	NT	NT	●	○	o
2.2	Unscheduled DNA synthesis (UDS)							
2.2.1		UDS in mouse liver	56	○	○	○	○	o
2.2.2		UDS in rat liver	56	○	○	●	○	o
2.2.3		UDS in rat liver	57	NT	NT	●	○	o
2.2.4		UDS in rat liver	58	○	○	●	○	o
2.2.5		UDS in mouse liver	58	NT	NT	○	○	o
2.2.6		UDS in rat liver	59	NT	NT	●	○	o
2.2.7		UDS in rat liver	60	NT	NT	●	○	o
2.2.8		UDS in rat liver	61	NT	NT	●	○	o
2.2.9		UDS in rat liver	62	NT	NT	●	○	o
2.2.10		UDS in weanling rat liver	63	○	NT	NT	NT	o
2.2.11		UDS - neonate rat	61	NT	NT	○	NT	o
2.3	S-phase hepatocytes							
2.3.1		Rat	56	○	NT	NT	●	o
2.3.2		Mouse	56	NT	NT	NT	○	o
2.3.3		Rat	58	○	○	●	●	o
2.3.4		Mouse	58	NT	NT	○	●	o
2.3.5		Rat	59	NT	NT	NT	●	o
2.3.6		Rat - weanling	63	●	NT	NT	NT	o
2.3.7		Rat	60	NT	NT	○	●	o
2.3.8		Rat	62	NT	NT	○	●	o
2.3.9		Rat	61	NT	NT	NT	●	o
2.4	Cytogenetic analysis							
2.4.1		Aberrations in liver epithelioid cells	65	○	○	○	C	o
2.4.2		SCE in liver epithelioid cells	65	○	○	?	○	o
2.4.3		Micronuclei in hepatocytes	66	○	○	●	○	o
2.5	DNA strand breaks							
2.5.1		Alkaline elution	68	○	○	○	○	o

Table 4 (contd.)

Assay		Chapter numbers[b]	BP	PYR	2AAF	4AAF	Route of exposure
2.5.2	Alkaline elution	69	○	○	◉	○	o
2.5.3	Alkaline elution	70	◉	○	◉	◉	o
2.5.4	DNA-DNA/DNA-protein crosslinks	70	◉	◉	◉	NT	ip
2.5.5	DNA unwinding	71	◉	◉	◉	○	o
2.5.6	DNA unwinding (with araA)	71	◉	○	◉	○	o

3. MISCELLANEOUS ASSAYS

3.1 Carcinogenesis

3.1.1	2-year rat study	73	NT	NT	◉	*	o
3.1.2	Mouse lung adenoma	74	◉	○	◉	○	o
3.1.3	Quail egg	75	*	*	*	*	

3.2 Supplementary assay

3.2.1	Rat fore-stomach UDS	76	?	○	○	○	o
3.2.2	Sebaceous gland suppression	77	◉	◉	NT	NT	der
3.2.3	Epithelial hyperplasia	77	◉	◉	NT	NT	der
3.2.4	Rat hepatocyte ploidy	78	◉	◉	◉	○	o
3.2.5	Mouse hepatocyte ploidy	78	◉	○	◉	○	o
3.2.6	Syrian hamster 6-TG-resistant lung cells	79	◉	○	?	○	ip
3.2.7a	^{32}P-post labelling - rat liver	80	◉	○	◉	○	ip
3.2.7b	^{32}P-post labelling - rat lung	80	◉	○	◉	○	ip
3.2.7c	^{32}P-post labelling - mouse liver	80	◉	○	◉	NT	ip
3.2.7d	^{32}P-post labelling - mouse lung	80	◉	○	◉	NT	ip
3.2.7e	^{32}P-post labelling - mouse kidney	80	◉	○	◉	NT	ip
3.2.8	Radiolabelled test compounds	81	NT	NT	◉	◉	ip
3.2.9	ELISA rat	82	NT	NT	*	*	o

3.3 Immunotoxicity

3.3.1	T-cells - rat	83	◉	○	◉	○	ip
3.3.2	Natural Killer cells - rat	84	NT	NT	◉	○	o

3.4 Transformation of peritoneal macrophages

3.4.1	Rat macrophages	85	○	○	○	○	o
3.4.2	Rat macrophages	85	○	○	○	○	o
3.4.3	Rat macrophages	85	○	○	○	○	o

3.5 Host-mediated assays

3.5.1a	Mouse/yeast - mitotic recombination - liver	86	NT	NT	○	○	o
3.5.1b	Mouse/yeast - mitotic recombination - lung	86	NT	NT	○	○	o

Assessment of the Performance of the Assays

Table 4 (contd.)

3.5.1c	Mouse/yeast - mitotic recombination - kidney	86	NT	NT	○	○		o
3.5.1d	Mouse/yeast - mutation - liver	86	NT	NT	○	○		o
3.5.1e	Mouse/yeast - mutation - lung	86	NT	NT	○	○		o
3.5.1f	Mouse/yeast - mutation - kidney	86	NT	NT	○	○		o
3.5.2a	Mouse/yeast - gene conversion - liver	87	●	●	●	●		o
3.5.2b	Mouse/yeast - gene conversion - lung	87	○	○	○	○		o
3.5.3	Mouse/salmonella - liver	88	○	○	○	○		o

3.6 Urine mutagenicity

3.6.1	Rat urine extract	89	●	●	●	●	ip
3.6.2	Rat urine extract	90	●	●	●	●	ip
3.6.3	Mouse urine extract	91	○	○	●	●	o
3.6.4a	Rat urine	92	●	●	●	●	ip
		92	●	●	●	●	o
3.6.4b	Guinea-pig	92	NT	NT	●	NT	ip
3.6.5	Rat urine	93	●	●	●	●	ip

4. MOUSE SPOT TEST

4.1.1	Coat color	95	NT	NT	●	○	ip
4.1.2	Coat color	96	NT	NT	○	○	o
		96	NT	NT	○	NT	ip
4.1.3	Coat color	97	●	○	●	○	ip
4.1.4	Melanocytes	98	NT	NT	●	?	ip
4.1.5	Melanocytes	99	NT	NT	○	○	ip

5. MAMMALIAN GERM CELL STUDIES

5.1 Dominant lethal

5.1.1	Female mice	102	●	○	○	○	ip
5.1.2	Male mice	103	●	○	○	○	ip
5.1.3	Male mice	104	●	○	○	○	ip
		104	○	?	NT	NT	o
5.1.4	Male mice	105	●	○	○	○	ip
		105	○	NT	NT	NT	o
5.1.5	Male rat	106	NT	NT	○	○	o

5.2 Sperm abnormalities

5.2.1	Mouse	108	●	○	●	○	ip
5.2.2	Mouse	109	○	○	○	○	o
5.2.3	Mouse	110	●	○	●	○	ip
5.2.4	Mouse	111	●	○	○	○	o
5.2.5	Rat	112	NT	NT	○	○	o

5.3 Unscheduled DNA synthesis

5.3.1	Rat spermatocytes	113	○	○	○	○	o

Evaluation of Short-term Tests for Carcinogens (In Vivo)

Table 4 (contd.)

Assay		Chapter numbers[b]	BP	PYR	2AAF	4AAF	Route of exposure
5.3.2	Mouse sperm	114	O	O	O	O	ip
		114	O	NT	NT	NT	o
6.	**DROSPHILA ASSAYS**						
6.1	Sex-linked recessive lethal						
6.1.1	SLRL assay	116	O	O	●	O	o
6.1.2	SLRL assay	117	O	O	O	O	o
6.1.3	SLRL assay	118	O	O	O	O	o
6.1.4	SLRL assay	119	O	O	O	O	o
6.1.5	SLRL assay	120	O	O	O	O	o
6.2	Chromosome loss						
6.2.1	Germ cell	121	O	O	O	O	o
6.2.2	Germ cell	116	O	NT	O	NT	o
6.3	Somatic mutation and recombination						
6.3.1	Eye spots	116	●	O	O	O	o
6.3.2	Eye spots	122	●	O	●	O	o
6.3.3	Wing spots	118	●	O	O	?	o

[a] From: Ashby et al. (1988)
[b] Numbers refer to chapters in Ashby et al. (1988)

● Positive   NT Not tested
O Negative   ? Inconclusive
o Weak positive   * Results not available

Assessment of the Performance of the Assays

8.1 Cytogenetic assays

Assays that utilize target cells in rodent bone marrow for detecting chromosomal effects, i.e., chromosomal aberrations, micronuclei, or sister chromatid exchanges, are widely advocated for investigating the activity of *in vitro* genotoxins in the intact animal and represent the largest group of tests in this study.

8.1.1 *Chromosomal aberrations*

Data from metaphase chromosome studies in mouse bone marrow were provided by seven investigators. Each investigator successfully discriminated between BP and PYR, and five sets of data determined 4AAF to be negative while two were inconclusive. The results of chromosome studies with 2AAF, however, were conflicting. Two laboratories identified 2AAF as a clastogen, one set of data were inconclusive and four investigators reported 2AAF as negative. There appears to be no simple explanation for these discrepancies, which were not associated with differences in mouse stain, route of treatment, sampling interval, or other aspects of experimental design. The mouse micronucleus assay (section 8.1.2) showed 2AAF to be an *in vivo* clastogen (though less potent than BP) and it is clear that the dosing schedules used in the metaphase chromosome assays were more than adequate to induce chromosome aberrations, i.e., 2AAF would be expected to be detected as a clastogen in the metaphase chromosome assay. One explanation for the negative findings in four laboratories may be the resolving power of the sample sizes used. Most standard protocols for the bone marrow metaphase assay require at least 50 cells per animal from 10 animals per dose/time group (i.e., 500 cells) to be analysed for aberrations at each data point. This recommended minimum figure was only achieved by three of the seven investigators and three others presented data on only 250 cells per dose/time group. These observations suggest that, with samples of this size, almost a 10-fold increase in aberrations over the control incidence would be required to demonstrate a significant induction of aberrations by 2AAF.

Two investigators conducted studies in Chinese hamster bone marrow cells. PYR was negative in both studies. In experiments in which 500 cells per dose/time group were analysed, BP and 2AAF were clearly positive while, when only 300 cells were used, the results were classified as weak positive with both carcinogens. It is interesting to note that 4AAF induced a weak positive response in Chinese hamster bone marrow in one study.

One set of data from rat bone marrow was presented and clearly separated BP from PYR. 2AAF, however, gave unambiguous data and 4AAF was negative.

The performance of the bone marrow cytogenetic assays did not, in general, meet the criteria for a reliable and reproducible short-term *in vivo* test. There are, however, serious reservations regarding the numbers of animals and the numbers of cells analysed in many of the studies and the results suggest that protocols designed to give an acceptable resolving power should be strictly adhered to..

1.2 *Micronuclei*

Eighteen laboratories conducted micronucleus tests; 16 laboratories performed assays on bone marrow cells from mice and two investigators used rats. Data were also presented on the incidence of micronuclei in circulating blood cells from adult and fetal mice.

Mouse bone marrow micronucleus assays were conducted to a common protocol with only minor deviations. At least 5 mice were used for each dose/time interval with 1000 cells being analysed from each animal. The data from these assays showed a high level of agreement between laboratories. Seventeen sets of data on BP were uniformly positive and 16 sets on PYR were negative. Similarly, 14 investigators showed 2AAF to be capable of inducing an increase in micronuclei and 4AAF was negative in 14 cases. There were only occasional anomalous results. For example, one laboratory failed to detect 2AAF, and another investigator recorded weak positive results from both PYR and 4AAF. These anomalies do not detract from the general accuracy and reproducibility of mouse micronucleus tests with the four test chemicals.

One investigator used erythrocytes from mouse peripheral blood to assay the incidence of micronuclei. The results were similar to those obtained in the bone marrow

Assessment of the Performance of the Assays

studies, i.e. BP and 2AAF were positive while PYR and 4AAF were considered to be negative by the criteria adopted for a positive response. In two laboratories, fetal blood was obtained from mice on day 15 of pregnancy, 30 or 48 h after oral dosing of the mother. BP was positive and PYR was negative in each of these studies. The fetal assay was less sensitive to the effects of 2AAF, one laboratory observing a small increase in micronuclei and the other finding no increase. 4AAF was inactive in fetal cells.

Two micronucleus studies were conducted in rat bone marrow cells and the results suggest that the response in the rat was weaker than that in the mouse. In one laboratory, 2AAF was positive and 4AAF negative; BP and PYR were not tested. The second investigator reported a positive response with BP and a negative one with PYR. This investigator's result with 2AAF is shown as positive in Table 4. However, using criteria decided by the micronucleus assay working group, it was concluded that 2AAF was negative in this assay. It was also considered that the protocol used in the rat studies was not designed for the optimum detection of micronuclei.

The results from the micronucleus tests confirm the value of the assay in mouse bone marrow as an accurate and reproducible means of qualitative discrimination between carcinogenic and non-carcinogenic chemicals.

8.1.3 Sister chromatid exchange

Nine investigators presented data on the induction of sister chromatid exchanges (SCE) *in vivo* using mice, rats, or Chinese hamsters. The test chemicals were administered by gavage or intraperitoneal injection and most investigators analysed SCE in bone marrow cells. One set of data were presented on SCE in mouse peripheral lymphocytes and another set on Chinese hamster intestinal epithelial cells. The two established carcinogens, BP and 2AAF, induced an increase in SCE in each of the six studies conducted in mouse bone marrow. In two of these studies, PYR induced a weak positive response and 4AAF was weakly positive in four of the six assays. Weak positive results were also obtained in rat bone marrow assays with the two presumed non-carcinogens, while BP and 2AAF were clearly positive. In experiments conducted in blood lymphocytes in mice and in bone marrow cells and intestinal epithelial cells in Chinese hamsters, BP and 2AAF gave positive results while PYR and 4AAF were negative. None of the experiments suggested that the route of administration of the test chemicals significantly influenced the qualitative results.

Both the established carcinogens were consistently positive in tests for the induction of SCE in three rodent species, suggesting that the SCE assay is a sensitive and reproducible *in vivo* test for genotoxic carcinogens. PYR or 4AAF, however, induced small (but significant) increases in the incidence of SCE in 8 of 22 tests, although the presumed non-carcinogens were much less potent inducers of SCE than their carcinogenic analogues. These observations raise a number of questions regarding the significance of small increases in SCE in *in vivo* tests. In the first instance, if 4AAF is confirmed to be non-carcinogenic in the current rodent bioassay, then these weak responses have to be regarded as 'false positives'. If, however, 4AAF is shown to have weak carcinogenic activity, then the weak positive responses obtained in four of the six mouse bone marrow studies can be interpreted as accurately reflecting the genotoxicity of 4AAF. In the report of the SCE Working Group (Tice et al., 1988) the biological relevance of statistically significant increases in SCE at unrealistically high doses was considered. It was suggested that multiple mechanisms are involved in the formation of SCE and that one of these may be a response to stress, either at the cell or animal level, caused by a toxic response to high doses of a chemical. The small induction of SCE observed after high doses of PYR or 4AAF, therefore, may not be related mechanistically to the larger increases in SCE seen after low doses of BP or 2AAF. Thus, the final assessment of the performance of the *in vivo* SCE assays depends, to a large extent, on the outcome of the 2-year bioassay with the AAF analogues, i.e. a negative result with 4AAF will cast serious doubts on the value of SCE tests for investigating the *in vivo* activity of *in vitro* genotoxins.

Assessment of the Performance of the Assays

8.2 Liver assays

The activity of certain genotoxic chemicals appears to be confined to the liver. Such chemicals do not, of course, induce detectable genetic changes in bone marrow cells or other extra-hepatic tissues and this has led to a need to develop techniques for investigating genotoxic or related changes in liver cells. The main thrust of this research has centred on the demonstration of unscheduled DNA synthesis in hepatocytes but data were also presented from a variety of other assays that used target cells in the liver.

8.2.1 Initiation and promotion

Two of the assays used in this group were specifically aimed at detecting initiating activity of the test chemicals. The chemicals were administered after partial hepatectomy, and the mice were then treated with the promotor, phenobarbital, for several weeks before liver sections were examined for the occurrence of pre-cancerous foci, i.e. groups of cells having elevated levels of the marker enzyme, *gamma*-glutamyl-transpeptidase (GGT). Both these protocols have been used successfully with many test chemicals and, in the present study, successfully separated BP and 2AAF from PYR and 4AAF. A third protocol was used to investigate the promoting activity of the test chemicals after initiation by pre-treatment with dimethylnitrosamine. This, too, successfully separated BP from PYR, but, although 2AAF produced an increase in GGT-positive foci, a weak positive response was also observed with 4AAF. The two other procedures used to study initiation/promotion events based on altered enzyme foci failed to detect BP in one assay and 2AAF in the second assay and are considered to be, primarily, research techniques and not yet suitable for routine application.

The two better-established assays showed quite clearly that both BP and 2AAF initiated altered enzyme foci in rat liver. The two presumed non-carcinogens were completely negative and these tests, although they cannot be regarded as "short-term" in the true sense, have a useful role in investigating liver carcinogenesis.

2.2 Unscheduled DNA synthesis and S-phase analysis

The investigators in this group used the detection of unscheduled DNA synthesis (UDS) as a measure of DNA repair initiated in response to chemical-induced damage to the DNA. In each study, UDS was detected using autoradiographic techniques that also allowed simultaneous measurement of S-phase cells, i.e. those cells undergoing normal DNA synthesis as a prelude to mitosis. Seven investigators examined 2AAF and 4AAF for the induction of UDS and S-phase cells in hepatocytes of male rats, and in two laboratories all four test chemicals were investigated in rats and mice. The induction of UDS and S-phase cells in rat fore-stomach was investigated in another laboratory. Although there were minor protocol variations, the UDS working group concluded that none of these significantly affected the results and there was excellent agreement in the observations and conclusions of the investigators.

2AAF was shown to be a potent inducer of UDS in rat hepatocytes and also caused proliferation of hepatic cells as shown by an increase in the number of cells in S-phase. In mice, however, 2AAF failed to induce SCE in either of two laboratories, though there was evidence of a weak induction of S-phase cells. Only low doses were examined, i.e. up to 50mg/kg, but the results indicate an important species difference in the response to 2AAF.

Administration of 4AAF to rats produced negative UDS results in four laboratories and weak positive results in three laboratories. Although the three weak positive results were initially determined without recourse to statistical analysis, a comprehensive analysis of the data by Margolin and Risko (1988) confirmed the initial interpretation. The six investigators who recorded the number of S-phase cells observed a marked increase in hepatic cell proliferation in rats dosed with 4AAF. This compound failed to induce UDS in mouse liver but did cause an increase in S-phase cells.

For comparative purposes, two laboratories also conducted UDS tests on hepatocytes *in vitro*. Both 2AAF and 4AAF induced UDS in rat hepatocytes but were negative in mouse cells.

Assessment of the Performance of the Assays

BP and PYR were tested in rats by two investigators and one assay was conducted in mice. Both chemicals failed to induce UDS in either species after oral dosing. In contrast, BP gave positive results in both rat and mouse hepatocytes treated *in vitro*.

In an investigation of the UDS activity of the four chemicals in rat fore-stomach, 2AAF, 4AAF, and PYR failed to induce UDS while BP gave equivocal results.

The performance of the UDS assay in rodents dosed with 2AAF or 4AAF is worthy of further consideration. 2AAF is a potent rat hepatocarcinogen and a potent inducer of UDS in rat hepatocytes. In the mouse, however, 2AAF did not induce UDS and, on balance, available data suggest that it does not produce liver tumours. Thus, for this chemical, the UDS results accurately reflect its hepatocarcinogenic potential. The current lack of cancer data on 4AAF precludes this kind of comparison, but the UDS data suggest that if 4AAF is carcinogenic, it is markedly less so than 2AAF.

Although fewer tests were conducted with BP and PYR, the data indicate that neither chemical induces UDS in rat or mouse liver, although BP was positive in *in vitro* UDS tests. The reason for this negative response to BP has an important bearing on the validity of the UDS assay for detecting potentially carcinogenic chemicals. Although BP is an established carcinogen, it has never been shown to produce tumours in rodent liver. There is sufficient evidence, however, to suggest that DNA-reactive adducts are formed in liver cells after dosing rodents with BP. For example, most of the data that show BP to be genotoxic *in vitro* are derived from tests in which metabolic activation is provided by an enzyme mixture derived from rat liver. In addition, BP clearly induces altered enzyme foci in rat liver, there is tentative evidence for the induction of DNA strand breakage based on DNA-DNA/DNA-protein crosslinks, and ^{32}P-post-labelling techniques indicate the presence of DNA adducts of BP metabolites in both rat and mouse liver. Therefore, although BP is not a hepatocarcinogen in rodents, there are data to suggest that (a) BP is metabolized in rodent liver to DNA-reactive metabolites, (b) interaction of DNA with BP metabolites does occur, and (c) based on data from the DNA unwinding test, some repair of the DNA lesions takes place. On this basis, the liver UDS assay should, theoretically, be capable of detecting BP-induced lesions in the liver. All these observations indicate that such factors as the distribution of BP to the liver after oral dosing, the rate of formation of genotoxic metabolites, the rate of detoxification, and the rate and nature of the DNA repair process yield an insufficient number of DNA adducts to produce a detectable UDS response.

In practice, of course, BP is easily detected in other *in vivo* tests such as those conducted in bone marrow cells. However, the results with BP and, to a lesser extent, 4AAF, suggest the need for additional evaluation of the performance of the *in vivo* UDS assay with liver-specific genotoxins.

2.3 DNA strand breaks

Data were considered from three different assay systems used to detect single-strand breaks in DNA. Results from the alkaline elution assay, in which two laboratories found no activity with any of the four test chemicals, indicate that this assay is of little value in investigating *in vivo* genotoxicity. The test for DNA-DNA/DNA-protein crosslinks and the DNA unwinding assay in rodent liver cells both gave very promising results and warrant further evaluation.

2.4 Cytogenetics

Three sets of data were considered in this group. Micronucleus assays were conducted in rat liver cells following partial hepatectomy. The results were similar to those obtained in the rat liver UDS assay, i.e. a dose-dependant response was obtained with 2AAF, while the remaining three chemicals gave negative results. The other two data sets were generated from analyses of chromosome aberrations and SCE in epithelial-like cells derived from weanling rat liver. Although the assays are relatively simple with clearly defined end-points, the results were either equivocal or negative and the sample sizes, i.e. the numbers of animals/cells per dose group, were too small to permit an effective assessment. Both

Assessment of the Performance of the Assays

the micronucleus test and the chromosome assays are worthy of further evaluation.

8.3 Miscellaneous assays

This section contains a wide variety of assays, some of which have been in use for many years while others, few of which were undertaken in more than one laboratory, are relatively new or in the process of development.

8.3.1 Specific carcinogenicity assays

Neither of the two procedures considered here can be regarded as short-term tests and final results from one of them, the assay in quail eggs, were not available at the time of the assessment. The results of the mouse adenoma assay, however, were available and showed a decisive discrimination between BP and PYR and a much smaller and less convincing difference between 2AAF and 4AAF.

8.3.2 Supplementary assays

Data from the sebaceous gland suppression test and the epidermal hyperplasia assay have shown a good correlation with skin carcinogenicity and have proved useful for comparing the carcinogenic potential of polycyclic hydrocarbons. Their value in this area was confirmed by the results of assays with BP and PYR but the application of these assays to other classes of chemicals is of uncertain value.

The hepatocytes of rodents include mono- and binucleated cells and nuclei that may be diploid, tetraploid, or octaploid. The ratio of cells with different levels of ploidy in liver varies with species and age and can be altered by exposure to certain chemicals. There have been references to the effects of various chemicals on liver ploidy ratios over a number of years, but there appears to be no consistent relationship between ploidy changes and chemical carcinogenesis. Thus the observation that the two carcinogens, BP and 2AAF, increase the ratio of diploid to tetraploid cells is of uncertain significance. The assay may be of value in studying liver cell kinetics but its value in the detection of *in vivo* genotoxicity is debatable.

The general principles of the *in vivo/in vitro* somatic mutation assay were developed in the late 1970's and showed initial promise as a test for investigating organ-specific mutations induced by chemical carcinogens. One investigator provided data from a modification of this technique in which cells isolated from lung tissue of treated Syrian hamsters were cultured *in vitro* and the induction of mutations was determined. A reproducible increase in mutations was observed in lung cells after dosing with BP, but the results with 2AAF and the two non-carcinogens were considered to be negative. Although this is a logical and potentially useful approach to studying *in vivo* genotoxicity, the method requires much wider evaluation before it can be considered as an acceptable assay.

The detection and identification of DNA adducts provides conclusive evidence that a metabolite of the administered chemical has interacted with one of the important target macromolecules of carcinogenesis. Theoretical considerations indicate that, for many chemical classes, the formation of DNA adducts is a prerequisite for permanent genetic changes, such as mutations, and for the initiation stage of carcinogenesis. Research has shown a direct relationship between the administered dose of a chemical and DNA-adduct formation, so that precise dosimetry in specific organs is possible. Three approaches were used in the study, though results from a novel technique using monoclonal antibodies to identify specific adducts are not yet available. One study involved the use of radiolabelled 2AAF and 4AAF; while binding to liver DNA was detected with both compounds, the covalent binding of 2AAF was approximately seven times that of 4AAF. These data correlate well with the results of the UDS assay in rat liver, which showed 2AAF to be a potent inducer of UDS while 4AAF was, at best, a weak inducer.

The above assay has the disadvantage of requiring radiolabelled test chemicals, and a significant advance in the field was the introduction of techniques in which animals are dosed with unlabelled test chemicals and the DNA is radiolabelled after isolation and purification. The

^{32}P-labelled normal nucleotides and nucleotide adducts are separated by thin-layer chromatography and detected by autoradiography, and a comprehensive, organospecific DNA adduct profile is obtained. The data presented in the current study showed that 2AAF adducts were detected at significant levels in the DNA of mouse liver, lung, and kidney and in rat liver and lung. 4AAF adducts were not detected in mouse tissue and at only very low levels in rat liver. PYR adducts were not detected in either rat or mouse tissues and BP produced adducts with DNA in liver and lung of both species and in mouse kidney.

The detection and identification of DNA adducts is potentially an extremely powerful tool in the investigation of *in vivo* genotoxicity. With the establishment of 'cold' techniques, i.e. those not requiring radiolabelled test chemicals, this type of assay can be applied to most chemical classes. Although further development is required, particularly with regard to the genotoxic significance of different types of adduct, the method shows great promise for the future.

8.3.3 Immunotoxicity assays

In the Natural Killer (NK) cell assay, the activity of NK cells was measured at intervals after dosing rats with either 2AAF or 4AAF. The carcinogen, 2AAF, induced a significant change in NK cell cytotoxicity that was not observed after dosing with 4AAF. The T-cell assay, in which immunocompetent T-cells are able to react to carcinogen-induced tissue changes, responded positively to BP and 2AAF; PYR failed to induce any change in reactivity and 4AAF gave a weak positive response. The results of both types of assay closely reflected the carcinogenic activity of the test chemicals. The relevance of the observed immunological changes to the carcinogenic process is unclear and, thus, their potential value in detecting precarcinogenic changes caused by genotoxic and non-genotoxic carcinogens remains to be fully evaluated. Before they can be accepted as anything more than a useful research tool, further investigations of the specificity of the immunological reactions and a wider evaluation are imperative.

3.4 Host-mediated assays and urine mutagenicity tests

As described at the beginning of Section 8, both these classes of test failed to meet the criteria for an acceptable short-term *in vivo* assay. The host-mediated assay was a favoured *in vivo* procedure in the early 1970s, though in recent years questions have been raised concerning its sensitivity. Although the intrasanguinous modification to the original intraperitoneal technique offered theoretical advantages, the results of the present study confirmed the inadequacy of the assay. It is concluded that both these procedures are not appropriate for the investigation of *in vitro* genotoxins.

4 Mouse spot tests

Although data were presented from two types of mouse spot test, they are, in effect, different means of observing the same genetic alterations, i.e. the melanocyte test detects the change at the cellular level while the coat colour test demonstrates the expression of the cellular changes.

BP and PYR were only tested in one laboratory and the spot test successfully identified the carcinogen. In tests with 4AAF, one investigator's results were considered to be inconclusive and four other sets of data, including one after oral dosing and three after intraperitoneal administration, were negative. Six laboratories tested 2AAF; there were three positive results and two negatives after intraperitoneal administration. 2AAF was also negative after oral dosing. Examination of the protocols indicated that 2AAF induced detectable genetic changes only after administration of the material as a solution in dimethylsulfoxide, i.e. negative results followed the administration of corn oil formulations of 2AAF, illustrating the critical effect of the vehicle on the absorption of the test chemical.

An overview of the mouse spot test data indicates that intraperitoneal administration of an appropriate formulation of the test chemicals produces results that reflect their carcinogenic activity. The original coat colour procedure appears to be more reliable than the melanocyte technique, which may be influenced by sporadic mutational events and inadequate melanization of the hair follicles. However, the dependence on the intraperitoneal route of administration may be a disadvantage, and the mouse spot test appears to add very little to the information gained more easily from bone marrow cell cytogenetic assays.

8.5 Assays in mammalian germ cells

For assessment purposes the germ cell assays have been separated into two groups: those that are considered to involve a direct interaction with DNA, and the assay for sperm abnormalities, the genetic significance of which is uncertain.

8.5.1 Dominant lethal and unscheduled DNA synthesis assays

Classical dominant lethal tests were conducted in male or female mice and in male rats. PYR, 2AAF, and 4AAF gave unequivocally negative results after intraperitoneal dosing. In an oral dosing study in male mice, BP was negative and PYR produced inconclusive data. After intraperitoneal administration of BP, however, there was conclusive evidence of dominant lethal induction in male and female mice. In the male, dominant lethality was confined to the late spermatid/spermatozoa stages of spermatogenesis.

Results of UDS assays in rat spermatocytes after oral dosing and in mouse spermatocytes after oral or intraperitoneal administration were negative with all four chemicals. The negative data with BP are not altogether surprising as dominant lethality was only observed in late spermatids/spermatozoa, in which the DNA is highly condensed and in which UDS does not occur.

Based on the dominant lethal test results, BP is a confirmed, though relatively weak, germ cell mutagen in mice after intraperitoneal dosing. Published data indicate that BP does not induce heritable translocations at doses that produce dominant lethality (Generoso et al., 1982), although this may be due, in part, to the fact that BP appears to induce mainly chromatid deletions in bone marrow cell chromosomes, with very few exchange-type aberrations.

5.2 Sperm abnormality tests

This assay is based on the observation of morphological alterations in mature spermatozoa after treatment of animals at all stages of spermatogenesis with the test chemicals. BP induced an increase in the incidence of abnormal sperm in mice after oral or intraperitoneal dosing and 2AAF was also positive following oral gavage. Tests with 4AAF were uniformly negative and PYR produced a weak positive response in one of four assays. Thus, both carcinogens produced sperm abnormalities under appropriate experimental conditions.

The important questions raised by these observations relate to the relevance of morphological abnormalities in sperm to germ cell mutations and to carcinogenesis. Although changes in sperm head shape may be genetically determined, it is uncertain whether they are due to genotoxicity or to other toxic phenomena. A positive result in the test, therefore, indicates that the test material or its metabolites are able to reach the germ cells in sufficient quantities to induce an adverse biological effect. Although a good correlation has been shown between the induction of sperm abnormalities and carcinogenic activity (Wyrobek et al., 1983), the relevance of this correlation to short-term testing strategies is doubtful as more appropriate *in vivo* tests are available, e.g., bone marrow cytogenetic assays. Equally doubtful is the relevance of the test to heritable genetic damage, as there is no clear-cut evidence that abnormal sperm are a consequence of induced DNA damage.

6 Drosophila assays

The sex-linked recessive lethal assay and the test for chromosome loss in drosophila germ cells failed to show a consistent separation of BP and 2AAF from PYR and 4AAF, respectively. Three tests based on somatic cell changes were positive with BP and negative with PYR but the results of tests with the acetylaminofluorenes were less decisive. 2AAF produced an unambiguous positive result and two weak positives, while the three results with 4AAF were weak positive, negative and inconclusive. Thus, the drosophila germ cell assays were insensitive to the four

Assessment of the Performance of the Assays

in vitro genotoxins and, although the somatic cell procedures appeared to be more sensitive, it was concluded that the main value of drosophila tests is to provide comprehensive analyses of the genetic mechanisms involved in the induction of mutations by chemicals.

9. SELECTION OF THE MOST EFFECTIVE *IN VIVO* ASSAYS IN RELATION TO THEIR PERFORMANCE

In a study of this nature it is inevitable that some assays, even well-established procedures, will fail to perform well. Indeed, the recognition of inadequate tests is as important a goal as the identification of those that are useful and acceptable. Other assays produced results that correlated well with the presumed carcinogenic status of the test chemicals but are not widely used or available or are still in the process of development. Yet other tests that performed adequately in the collaborative study cannot be regarded as practicable short-term tests either because of their technical complexity or because of the length of time required to produce results. Most of the latter group of tests have important research roles in carcinogenesis.

1 **Assays that are not considered appropriate for routine *in vivo* testing of chemicals for genotoxic activity**

Host-mediated and urine mutagenicity assays (section 8.3.4), the peritoneal macrophage transformation assay, and the alkaline elution assay for single strand breaks (section 8.2.3) proved incapable of separating the carcinogen/non-carcinogen pairs and appear to have little value in investigating *in vivo* genotoxicity. The *in vivo/in vitro* somatic mutation procedure in Syrian hamsters (section 8.3.2) also falls into this category, although this conclusion should not detract from the initial promise of this approach in Chinese hamsters (McGregor, 1988a).

Drosophila tests (section 8.6) have also proved generally inadequate in the identification of *in vivo* genotoxins and it is concluded that their main value in genetic toxicology is to provide analysis of the genetic mechanisms involved in the induction of mutations. Similar reservations apply to the initiation/promotion techniques using liver foci (section 8.2.1) and the analysis of ploidy levels in liver tissue (section 8.3.2). Both assays are more appropriate to investigation of the carcinogenic process than to the identification of *in vivo* genotoxins. The results of the immunological assays (section 8.3.3) closely reflected the carcinogenic potential of the chemicals, but they can only be regarded as research tools pending a greater understanding of the specificity of the immunological reactions and a wider evaluation of the procedures.

Two assays conducted in mouse skin, i.e. the sebaceous gland suppression test and the observation of epidermal hyperplasia, confirmed their value in the detection of carcinogenic polycyclic hydrocarbons such as BP. Both tests failed to respond to 2AAF when applied dermally and are not considered to be suitable for investigating *in vivo* genotoxicity in general.

9.2 Assays that satisfy some or all of the criteria for an acceptable short-term *in vivo* test

9.2.1 Assays currently in general use

The mouse micronucleus test (section 8.1.2) was the most widely represented single assay in the study and produced the best overall performance with only occasional anomalous data. Qualitative results were not affected significantly by the route of exposure, strain or sex of mouse, or treatment schedule. The mouse bone marrow micronucleus assay was confirmed as a robust and sensitive short-term *in vivo* test for genotoxic chemicals.

Both the micronucleus test and the analysis of metaphase chromosome aberrations in rodent bone marrow respond to similar chromosome breakage events and they would be expected to produce qualitatively similar results with the four test compounds. Table 4 shows that this was not the case and the metaphase chromosome procedure was significantly less sensitive than the micronucleus test. Possible explanations for this lack of sensitivity are discussed above (section 8.1.1) and suggest that the use of metaphase chromosome analysis should not be undervalued on the basis of these data.

The sister chromatid exchange (SCE) procedure reproducibly detected the two carcinogens, but also produced a number of weak positive results with 4AAF and PYR. Taken at face value, therefore, the *in vivo* SCE results clearly reflect the relative potency of the two chemical pairs in *in vitro* tests. As discussed in section 8.1.3, however, very weak SCE responses may be caused by non-genotoxic mechanisms and a final judgement on the significance of the weak activity of 4AAF must be delayed until its true carcinogenic status is defined.

After considering the data from the three classes of bone marrow assay, the conclusion of the Steering Group (Ashby et al., 1988) was - 'the mouse micronucleus assay provides the simplest and most effective measure of genotoxicity in the bone marrow and, as such, it is recommended here as a primary *in vivo* genotoxicity test'.

Despite the successful performance of the micronucleus test with these four chemicals, it is apparent from the literature that certain liver carcinogens do not induce detectable chromosomal effects in the bone marrow. In an acceptable testing strategy, therefore, negative results in the micronucleus test should be supplemented with evidence of non-genotoxicity in the liver. This concept led to the extensive evaluation of liver-specific assays in the CSSTT/2 study and the main candidate in this group of tests was the rat liver UDS assay (section 8.2.2).

The liver carcinogen, 2AAF, was a potent inducer of UDS in rat liver while most investigators defined its presumed non-carcinogenic analogue, 4AAF, as a weak genotoxin in this system. Unlike the micronucleus test result, BP was devoid of activity in liver UDS assays. This is consistent with its lack of carcinogenicity in rat liver.

Although the significance of the weak liver UDS activity of 4AAF will only be resolved when definitive carcinogenicity data are available, the findings raise certain problems of interpretation that are common, in part, to the weak bone marrow activity of 4AAF and PYR. In the UDS assays, 2AAF was a potent inducer of UDS at doses between 5 and 100 mg/kg while 4AAF showed only weak activity between 50 and 1000 mg/kg, and then only in some experiments. In general, the activity of 4AAF was within the range of control variability and, as a result, the UDS Working Group questioned its biological significance

(Mirsalis, 1988). A detailed analysis, however, indicated the high statistical significance of the 4AAF data (Margolin and Risko, 1988). Thus, although the rat liver UDS assay discriminated quantitatively between 2AAF and 4AAF, the significance of the weak activity of 4AAF remains unresolved. These observations suggest that qualitative determinations in terms of 'positive' and 'negative' are too simplistic for hazard assessment purposes and one of the most useful points raised by the present study is the need for appropriate positive test criteria, in biological and statistical terms, for widely used *in vivo* tests.

Thus, the mouse bone marrow micronucleus assay is the method of choice for primary *in vivo* testing of *in vitro* genotoxins and the rat liver UDS assay, providing the above problems can be resolved, appears to be the most promising complementary liver-specific test.

9.2.2 Assays that show promise for future development

Accepting that bone marrow assays are suitable for detecting extra-hepatic somatic cell genotoxins and that the rat liver UDS assay can, with certain reservations (see sections 8.2.2 and 9.2.1), be used to investigate liver-specific genotoxins, it is useful to consider which other assays evaluated in this study may have a role in the assessment of *in vivo* genotoxicity.

Development of assays to detect single-strand breaks in DNA and to detect and identify DNA adducts will, undoubtedly, continue. It will be interesting to follow the progress of the assays for DNA-DNA/DNA-protein cross-links and DNA unwinding, although it is probable that their technical complexity will limit widespread use and acceptance. Of the DNA adduct techniques represented, the post-labelling method appears to hold most promise. The need for radiolabelled test compounds or specific monoclonal antibodies is eliminated and the assay provides information on the direct interaction of test chemicals with DNA in a variety of target organs, including the liver. Providing a reliable and robust protocol can be established and pending the provision of more information regarding the relationship between DNA adduct formation and genotoxic changes to the DNA, this assay could have an important role to play in the assessment of genotoxic hazard.

The performance of the cytogenetic assays in liver cells was disappointing but, theoretically, they could, with further development, prove to be of value in the assessment of liver-specific genotoxicity. The reliance of the current micronucleus procedure on partial hepatectomy is a disadvantage, but the development of alternative means of stimulating hepatic mitotic activity, either *in vivo* or in short-term culture, could be the basis of a useful short-term liver-specific assay. Cytogenetic assays on circulating blood cells performed reasonably well and the theoretical and practical advantages of tests for SCE or micronuclei in circulating blood should encourage further development of these tests.

The mouse spot test, in its original form (section 6.4), successfully separated the carcinogen/non-carcinogen pairs and, providing care is taken in the selection of an appropriate solvent or formulation, it appears to be a useful and reproducible assay. Its availability is limited by the need to maintain specific mouse strains and its overall sensitivity, compared to the micronucleus test, is suspect, as positive results in the present study were dependant on intraperitoneal dosing.

3 The detection of germ cell mutagens

The performance and significance of the three germ cell assays represented in the study are discussed above (section 8.5). Only BP was clearly identified as a germ cell mutagen in the dominant lethal assay. The failure of the sperm abnormality test to discriminate between BP and 2AAF suggests that this assay is affected by non-genetic toxic effects and is, therefore, of doubtful value in predicting the induction of mutations in mammalian germ cells.

Although there are theoretical reasons why BP should not induce UDS in germ cells (section 8.5.1), this negative result raises questions similar to those resulting from the failure of BP to induce UDS in rat liver (section 8.2.2), i.e. why does BP not induce detectable UDS in target cells where there is evidence, from other assays, of genotoxic activity?

As concluded by Ashby et al. (1988) 'the germ cell activities of BP have served to focus several important, but unresolved, issues associated with the conduct of, and the interpretation of data derived from, germ cell genotoxicity and mutagenicity assays'.

9.4 Influence of the route of administration of the test chemicals

A feature of the micronucleus assays was that their qualitative separation of BP and 2AAF from PYR and 4AAF was not influenced by the route of administration of the chemicals. Dominant lethal mutations, however, were only detected after intraperitoneal dosing with BP; oral dosing was ineffective. Similarly, the mouse spot test was dependant on the intraperitoneal route of administration for the demonstration of mutagenic effects. The introduction of the test material in the vicinity of the uterus in the spot test circumvents the natural pharmacokinetics and metabolic routes of the test animal, and it can be argued that this unrealistic pattern of exposure does not reflect true *in vivo* genotoxicity. It can be similarly argued that the purpose of *in vivo* tests is to achieve maximum exposure of the target cells and that intraperitoneal dosing can be justified for this reason. It may be, as suggested by Shelby (1986), that intraperitoneal dosing should be reserved for assays used in a screening mode, i.e. for the detection of genotoxic activity, and that for investigating the *in vivo* activity of established genotoxins, a route of administration should be chosen that reflects possible human exposure. Arguments such as these must be resolved before strategies for testing chemicals for genotoxic activity can be fully harmonized.

10. CONCLUSIONS

Of the fifty or so separate *in vivo* techniques represented in the CSSTT/2 study, only a small number satisfied the criteria defined for an acceptable short-term *in vivo* test (section 3.2). These criteria, however, defined a very specific purpose, i.e. the identification of *in vivo* activity of established *in vitro* genotoxins. In order to generate a comprehensive data base on the four test chemicals, assays included in the study were not limited to, for example, those that were considered most likely to meet the criteria. As a result, some investigators submitted data from assays that were not designed for detecting *in vivo* genotoxins but, nevertheless, provided valuable information on a broad spectrum of biological effects of the test chemicals. The failure of such tests to satisfy the narrow selection criteria used in CSSTT/2 should not be regarded as a reflection on the validity of the procedures for specific research purposes. With these considerations in mind, and based on the concept (section 3.2) that short-term assays are required to investigate both liver-specific and extra-hepatic genotoxicity, the following conclusions appear appropriate.

1. Most of the *in vivo* somatic cell assays for genotoxicity were able to discriminate between the two carcinogen/non-carcinogen pairs, although, in some instances, weak activity was observed in tests with the non-carcinogens, particularly with 4AAF.

2. The weak genotoxicity of 4AAF in some studies suggested that qualitative determinations in terms of 'positive' and 'negative' are too simplistic for hazard assessment purposes and highlights the need for appropriate positive test criteria, in biological and statistical terms, for widely used *in vivo* tests.

3. The insensitivity of some assays to one or other of the two pairs of compounds supports the concept that negative *in vivo* data should be produced from at least two assays in different tissues, i.e. one in extra-hepatic somatic tissues and one in the liver, if they are to be used for assessing genotoxic hazard.

Conclusions

4. The mouse bone marrow micronucleus test was confirmed as a robust and sensitive assay and is the assay of choice for primary *in vivo* testing of *in vitro* genotoxins.

5. The overall performance of the rat liver UDS assay suggests that it could be complementary to the micronucleus test providing the reservations raised above (sections 8.2.2 and 9.2.1) can be satisfied. Development and evaluation of alternative procedures for investigating liver genotoxicity should be actively pursued.

6. Certain widely advocated assays, including the host-mediated and urine mutation assays and tests using drosophila are concluded to be inappropriate for hazard-assessment purposes.

7. BP and 2AAF showed genotoxic activity in the organs in which they also produce tumours. Their genotoxic activity in other tissues, however, precludes the use of data from short-term tests for making predictions of organ-specific carcinogenicity.

8. The majority of the positive responses observed in this study were obtained after oral administration of the test chemicals and at doses substantially below lethal levels, suggesting that short-term *in vivo* assays are not intrinsically insensitive, as is sometimes inferred. Positive results were obtained in the dominant lethal assay and the mouse spot test after intraperitoneal dosing only; both assays produced negative results after oral administration. These facts suggest that the intraperitoneal route should be reserved for the detection of genotoxic activity and that, for hazard-assessment purposes, a route of administration should be chosen that is relevant to the perceived route(s) of human exposure.

9. The germ cell mutagenicity exhibited by BP was adequately predicted by the somatic cell mutagenicity assays, adding weight to the suggestion that tests on mammalian germ cells should only be conducted to gain further information on the mutagenic spectrum of established *in vivo* somatic cell mutagens.

10. The occurrence of chemical carcinogens that fail to show evidence of genotoxicity in *in vitro* and *in vivo* assays indicates the existence of a class of chemicals that induce cancer by a mechanism that is not a conse-

quence of a direct interaction with DNA. The acceptance of the validity of the concept of non-genotoxic mechanisms of cancer induction is considered to be a crucial question in the future deployment of short-term tests in carcinogenesis.

11. The overall conclusion from the CSSTT/2 study is that short-term *in vivo* tests have a vital role to play in hazard assessment. This role is to define which chemicals, identified as genotoxic from *in vitro* tests, are active *in vivo* and, thus, are those most likely to present a carcinogenic/mutagenic hazard to mammals, including humans.

References

ASHBY, J., DE SERRES, F.J., DRAPER, M., ISHIDATE, M., Jr, MARGOLIN, B.H., MATTER, B., & SHELBY, M.D., ed. (1985) *Evaluation of short-term tests for carcinogens,* Amsterdam, Oxford, New York, Elsevier Science Publishers (Progress in Mutation Research, Vol. 5).

ASHBY, J., DE SERRES, F.J., SHELBY, M.D., MARGOLIN, B.H., ISHIDATE, M., Jr, & BECKING, G.C., ed. (1988a) *Evaluation of short-term tests for carcinogens: Report of the International Programme on Chemical Safety's collaborative study on in vivo assays,* Cambridge, United Kingdom, Cambridge University Press, Vol. 1.

ASHBY, J., SHELBY, M.D., & DE SERRES, F.J. (1988b) Overview of the IPCS collaborative study on *in vivo* assay systems and conclusions. In: Ashby, J., de Serres, F.J., Shelby, M.D., Margolin, B.H., Ishidate, M., Jr, & Becking, G.C., ed. *Evaluation of short-term tests for carcino-gens: Report of the International Programme on Chemical Safety's collaborative study on in vivo assays,* Cambridge, United Kingdom, Cambridge University Press, Vol. 1, pp. 6-28.

DE SERRES, F.J. & ASHBY, J., ed. (1981) *Evaluation of short-term tests for carcinogens: Report of the international collaborative study,* Amsterdam, Oxford, New York, Elsevier Science Publishers (Progress in Mutation Research, Vol. 1).

GENEROSO, W.M., CAIN, K.T., HELLWIG, C.S. & CACHEIRO, N.L.A. (1982) Lack of association between induction of dominant-lethal mutations and induction of heritable translocations with benzo(a)pyrene in postmeiotic germ cells of male mice. *Mutat. Res.,* **94**: 155-163.

HICKS, M.R., ASHBY, J., & PENMAN, M. (1988) Review of the rodent carcinogenicity data for the four test chemicals. In: Ashby, J., de Serres, F.J., Shelby, M.D., Margolin, B.H., Ishidate, M., Jr, & Becking, G.C., ed. *Evaluation of short-term tests for carcinogens: Report of the International Programme on Chemical Safety's collaborative study on in vivo assays,* Cambridge, United Kingdom, Cambridge University Press, Vol. 2, pp. 351-365.

MCGREGOR, D. (1988a) Summary report on the performance of the miscellaneous group of *in vivo* assays (carcinogenicity, DNA adducts, immunological, host-mediated mutation, urinary mutation assays, and limited metabolic assays. In: Ashby, J., de Serres, F.J., Shelby, M.D., Margolin, B.H., Ishidate, M., Jr, & Becking, G.C., ed. *Evaluation of short-term tests for carcinogens: Report of the International Programme on Chemical Safety's collaborative study on in vivo assays,* Cambridge, United Kingdom, Cambridge University Press, Vol. 2, pp. 3-21.

MCGREGOR, D. (1988b) The activities of 2AAF, 4AAF, BP and PYR in *in vitro* assays for genetic toxicity. In: Ashby, J., de Serres, F.J., Shelby, M.D., Margolin, B.H., Ishidate, M., Jr, & Becking, G.C., ed. *Evaluation of short-term tests for carcinogens: Report of the International Programme on Chemical Safety's collaborative study on in vivo assays,* Cambridge, United Kingdom, Cambridge University Press, Vol. 2, pp. 345-350.

MARGOLIN, B.H. & RISKO, K.J. (1988) The statistical analysis of *in vivo* genotoxicity data: case studies of the rat hepatocyte UDS and mouse bone marrow micronucleus assays. In: Ashby, J., de Serres, F.J., Shelby, M.D., Margolin, B.H., Ishidate, M., Jr, & Becking, G.C., ed. *Evaluation of short-term tests for carcinogens: report of the International Programme on Chemical Safety's collaborative study on in vivo assays,* Cambridge, United Kingdom, Cambridge University Press, Vol. 1, pp. 29-42.

MIRSALIS, J.C. (1988) Summary report on the performance of the *in vivo* DNA repair assays. In: Ashby, J., de Serres, F.J., Shelby, M.D., Margolin, B.H., Ishidate, M., Jr, & Becking, G.C., ed. *Evaluation of short-term tests for carcinogens: Report of the International Programme on Chemical Safety's collaborative study on in vivo assays,* Cambridge, United Kingdom, Cambridge University Press, Vol. 1, pp. 345-351.

PATON, D. & ASHBY, J. (1988) Source and analytical details of the test chemicals. In: Ashby, J., de Serres, F.J., Shelby, M.D., Margolin, B.H., Ishidate, M., Jr, & Becking, G.C., ed. *Evaluation of short-term tests for carcinogens: Report of the International Programme on Chemical Safety's collaborative study on in vivo assays,* Cambridge, United Kingdom, Cambridge University Press, Vol. 2, pp. 341-344.

SHELBY, M.D. (1986) A case for the continued use of the intraperitoneal route of exposure. *Mutat. Res.,* 70: 169-171.

TICE, R.R. (1988) Summary report on the performance of the *in vivo* sister chromatid exchange assays. In: Ashby, J., de Serres, F.J., Shelby, M.D., Margolin, B.H., Ishidate, M., Jr, & Becking, G.C., ed. *Evaluation of short-term tests for carcinogens: Report of the International Programme on Chemical Safety's collaborative study on in vivo assays,* Cambridge, United Kingdom, Cambridge University Press, Vol. 1, pp. 233-253.

WHO (1985) Environmental Health Criteria 47: Summary report on the evaluation of short-term tests for carcinogens (collaborative study on *in vitro* tests), Geneva, World Health Organization, 77 pp.

WYROBEK, A.J., GORDON, L.A., BURKHART, J.G., FRANCIS, M.W., KAPP, R.W., LETZ, G., MALLING, H.V., TOPHAM, J.C., & WHORTON, M.D. (1983) An evaluation of the mouse sperm morphology test and other tests in non-human mammals: A report of the United States Environmental Protection Agency Gene-Tox Program. *Mutat. Res.,* 115: 1-7.

RESUME

ETUDE COLLECTIVE DU PROGRAMME INTERNATIONAL SUR LA SECURITE DES SUBSTANCES CHIMIQUES (IPCS) POUR L'EVALUATION ET LA VALIDATION DES EPREUVES DE COURTE DUREE RELATIVES AUX CANCEROGENES

La première partie de ce projet, qui traite des études *in vitro*, a été publiée en 1985 (Ashby et al., 1985); on en trouvera un résumé dans le No 47 de la série Critères d'hygiène de l'environnement (OMS 1985). La seconde partie, qui fait l'objet du présent rapport, a été publieé en 1988 (Ashby et al., 1988).

Devant la nécessité d'évaluer l'intérêt des épreuves de courte durée pour la recherche des substances mutagènes et cancérogènes, il devenait indispensable d'organiser des études collectives inter-laboratoires à l'échelle internationale. Ces épreuves de courte durée devaient compléter les épreuves classiques à long terme sur rongeurs ou s'y substituer. C'est le problème du choix ainsi que de la fiabilité et de la sensibilité de ces épreuves qui a conduit à la première grande entreprise de collaboration au niveau international, à savoir le Programme coopératif international pour l'évaluation des épreuves de courte durée relatives aux cancérogènes (IPESTTC) (de Serres & Ashby, 1981). Les résultats de cette étude ont confirmé la fiabilité et la faisabilité de l'épreuve de mutation des salmonelles pour une première identification des substances cancérogènes et mutagènes. On a également constaté qu'avec cette épreuve, certains produits notoirement cancérogènes chez les rongeurs étaient impossibles ou tout du moins très difficiles à mettre en évidence. Un certain nombre d'autres épreuves examinées dans le cadre de l'étude IPESTTC se sont révélées capables de mettre en évidence quelques-uns des cancérogènes murins pour lesquels l'épreuve sur salmonelle donnait un résultat négatif. Toutefois, la base de données était trop restreinte pour qu'on puisse recommander une épreuve capable de compléter l'épreuve de mutation des salmonelles.

Au vu des résultats de l'étude IPESTTC, il est apparu nécessaire de poursuivre ce type de coopération afin d'établir a) quel est l'ensemble d'épreuves *in vitro* le plus efficace pour un premier tri des substances chimiques sur la base de leur activité génotoxique et b) quelles sont les épreuves *in vivo* de courte durée les plus utiles pour confirmer la génotoxicité et le pouvoir cancérogène des substances chimiques chez les mammifères. L'étude collective pour l'évaluation et la validation des épreuves de génotoxicité et de cancérogénicité de courte durée (CSSTT), a été proposée par le Programme international sur la sécurité des substances chimiques (IPCS) et le National Institute of Environmental Health Sciences (NIEHS) des Etats-Unis d'Amérique, l'une des institutions qui participent au Programme IPCS. Devant l'ampleur de cette entreprise et du fait des problèmes logistiques que posent l'organisation et la gestion de ce genre d'études internationales, le projet a été divisé en deux études distinctes: l'Etude collective sur les épreuves de génotoxicité et de cancérogénicité de courte durée *in vitro* (CSSTT/1) et l'Etude collective sur les épreuves de mutagénicité et de cancérogénicité de courte durée *in vivo* (CSSTT/2).

L'Etude CSSTT/1 a permis de constituer une vaste base de données à partir d'épreuves *in vitro* très diverses portant sur dix produits chimiques organiques. Parmi eux figuraient huit substances de cancérogénicité reconnue pour les rongeurs qui s'étaient révélées soit négatives à l'épreuve sur salmonelle soit difficiles à reconnaître de cette manière, ainsi que deux substances considérées comme non cancérogènes. On a procédé à l'évaluation de données tirées de 90 groupes d'épreuves effectuées par quelque 60 scientifiques. Quatre types d'épreuves ont donné des résultats suffisamment bons pour qu'on puisse envisager de les utiliser en complément à l'épreuve sur salmonelle. Il s'agissait de la recherche des aberrations chromosomiques, des mutations géniques et des transformations néoplasiques en culture de cellules mammaliennes ainsi que de l'épreuve d'aneuploïdie des levures. Sauf dans le cas de la recherche des aberrations chromosomiques, on a constaté que les protocoles généralement utilisés pour ces épreuves devaient être étudiés plus à fond avant d'être considérés comme tout à fait acceptables.

Resumé

La principale conclusion de l'étude CSSTT/1 relative aux épreuves *in vitro*, c'est que en combinant l'épreuve de recherche des aberrations chromosomiques à l'épreuve de mutation des salmonelles, on peut procéder à un premier criblage efficace des substances cancérogènes.

Lors de l'étude IPESTTC, sept substances sur 14 supposées non cancérogènes ont donné des résultats positifs dans un grand nombre d'épreuves *in vitro*. D'après les données *in vivo* limitées qu'a fournies cette étude, il semblerait que ces sept produits soient inactifs dans les épreuves de courte durée *in vivo*. Les produits non cancérogènes de deux des couples cancérogène/non-cancérogène soumis à l'étude IPESTTC, à savoir le couple benzo[a]pyrène/pyrène (BP/PYR) et le couple acétyl-2 aminofluorène/acétyl-4 aminofluorène (2AAF/4AAF), constituent de bons exemples de ces réactions différentes et d'ailleurs, ces couples de produits avaient été retenus pour la partie *in vivo* de l'étude collective (CSSTT/2). Toutefois, il y avait doute quant à la non cancérogénicité supposée du 4AAF et une part très importante de l'étude a été consacrée à la mise en route d'études de cancérogéniticé à long terme sur le 2AAF et le 4AAF chez le rat.

L'objectif de l'étude CSSTT/2 était donc de produire un profil de données complet à partir d'une large gamme d'épreuve *in vivo* de courte durée afin de voir comment les différents paramètres génétiques des tissus-cibles se comportent vis-à-vis de produits chimiques classés comme génotoxiques d'après les épreuves *in vitro*. La finalité de l'étude était de recenser les épreuves *in vivo* susceptibles d'être utilisées pour déterminer l'activité *in vivo* de substances notoirement génotoxiques.

Quatre-vingt-dix-sept chercheurs de 16 pays ont participé à l'étude *in vivo*, les données présentées portant sur une cinquantaine de techniques distinctes. Les résultats ont été évalués lors d'une réunion de ces chercheurs qui s'est tenue au Cap d'Agde (France) en mai 1985. On a préparé une série de rapports comportant une évaluation de chaque groupe d'épreuves, des rapports récapitulatifs sur les épreuves relatives aux cellules germinales et les épreuves d'hépatotoxicité et des rapports résumant toute la base de données relative à chaque couple de produits.

Par la suite, on a préparé un récapitulatif de toute l'étude *in vivo* en vue de sa publication définitive.

Seule une faible proportion des épreuves examinées lors de l'étude CSSTT/2 ont satisfait aux critères d'acceptabilité comme épreuves *in vivo* de courte durée. Toutefois les épreuves examinées lors de cette étude ne se limitaient pas à celles jugées a priori les plus conformes aux critères. De la sorte, on a pu tirer des données provenant d'épreuves qui, à l'origine, n'étaient pas des épreuves de génotoxicité *in vivo*, des renseignements sur une large gamme d'effets biologiques produits par ces quatre substances. La plupart des épreuves de génotoxicité *in vivo* portant sur des cellules somatiques permettaient de distinguer les deux couples cancérogène/non-cancérogène encore que dans certains cas, les produits non cancérogènes, en particulier le 4AAF aient présenté une faible activité. L'insensibilité de certaines épreuves à l'un ou à l'autre des deux couples de produits chimiques, corroborent l'idée selon laquelle il faut obtenir des résultats négatifs *in vivo* dans au moins deux épreuves pratiquées sur des tissus différents avant de considérer qu'un produit chimique n'est pas génotoxique *in vivo*.

Il a été confirmé que l'épreuve des micro-noyaux sur moëlle osseuse de souris est robuste, sensible et reproductible et on la recommande pour une première recherche de la génotoxicité *in vivo* et *in vitro*. Les résultats généraux obtenus au moyen de l'épreuve sur foie de rat pour la synthèse anarchique de l'ADN incitent à penser qu'elle pourrait compléter l'épreuve des micro-noyaux, mais il faut en étudier encore la sensibilité et la sélectivité. Certaines épreuves pourtant largement préconisées, notamment les épreuves par passage sur hôte, les épreuves de mutagénicité des urines et les épreuves sur drosophile, se sont révélées impropres à une évaluation du risque.

Les résultats de l'étude CSSTT/2 ont confirmé que les épreuves *in vivo* de courte durée ont un rôle capital à jouer dans l'évaluation du risque, rôle qui consiste dans l'identification des produits chimiques qui s'étant révélés génotoxiques *in vitro*, sont également actifs *in*

Resumé

vivo et comportent donc vraisemblablement un risque de cancérogénicité ou de mutagénicité pour les mammifères en général et l'homme en particulier.

RESUMEN

PROGRAMA INTERNACIONAL DE SEGURIDAD DE LAS SUSTANCIAS QUIMICAS (IPCS): ESTUDIO EN COLABORACION SOBRE EVALUACION Y COMPROBACION DE PRUEBAS A CORTO PLAZO PARA SUSTANCIAS CARCINOGENAS

La primera parte del presente proyecto, relativa a estudios *in vitro*, se publicó en 1985 (Ashby et al., 1985) y se resumió en la publicación 47 de la serie "Environmental Health Criteria" (OMS, 1985). La segunda parte es el tema del presente informe y se publicó en 1988 (Ashby et al., 1988).

La necesidad de estudios en colaboración entre laboratorios en escala internacional surgió de que era imprescindible investigar el valor de las pruebas a corto plazo para detectar las sustancias químicas mutágenas y carcinógenas. Se propusieron los ensayos a corto plazo como métodos que sustituyeran o complementaran a los tradicionales ensayos biológicos a largo plazo en roedores. La preocupación por la elección de las pruebas a corto plazo y por su fiabilidad y sensibilidad condujo a que se realizara el primer ejercicio importante de colaboración internacional: el programa internacional en colaboración sobre evaluación de las pruebas a corto plazo para sustancias carcinógenas (IPESTTC) (de Serres y Ashby, 1981). Los resultados de ese estudio confirmaron el valor de la prueba de mutación de salmonelas como ensayo fiable y factible para la identificación primaria de sustancias carcinógenas y mutágenas. Se observó también que en la prueba de salmonelas no se detectaban o sólo se detectaban con grandes dificultades algunas sustancias de cancerogenicidad conocida en los roedores. Otros ensayos incluidos en el estudio IPESTTC pudieron detectar sustancias carcinógenas para roedores que eran negativas en el ensayo de salmonelas. Sin embargo, la base de datos de apoyo era demasiado pequeña para permitir la recomendación de un ensayo que complementara la prueba de mutación de salmonelas.

Los resultados del estudio IPESTTC pusieron de manifiesto que se necesitaría un nuevo ejercicio en

Resumen

colaboración para determinar: a) la combinación más eficaz de ensayos *in vitro* para la detección primaria de la actividad genotóxica de sustancias químicas, y b) las pruebas *in vivo* a corto plazo más útiles para confirmar la posibilidad de genotoxicidad y cancerogenicidad en mamíferos. El Programa Internacional sobre Seguridad de las Sustancias Químicas (IPCS) y el Instituto Nacional de Ciencias de Higiene del Medio (NIHS) de los Estados Unidos de América, como institución participante en el IPCS, propusieron el estudio en colaboración sobre evaluación y comprobación de las pruebas a corto plazo para la genotoxicidad y la cancerogenicidad (CSSTT). Dadas la magnitud prevista del proyecto y la logística de la organización y administración de los proyectos internacionales, el proyecto se dividió en dos estudios independientes: el estudio en colaboración sobre pruebas a corto plazo para la genotoxicidad y la cancerogenicidad (CSSTT/1) y el estudio en colaboración sobre pruebas in vivo a corto plazo para sustancias mutágenas y carcinógenas (CSSTT/2).

En el estudio CSSTT/1 se reunió una abarcante base de datos procedentes de una amplia gama de ensayos *in vitro* realizados con diez productos químicos orgánicos cuidadosamente seleccionados. Incluían ocho sustancias de cancerogenicidad probada para roedores, que resultaban negativas o difíciles de detectar en el ensayo de salmonelas y dos sustancias químicas consideradas como no carcinógenas. Se evaluaron los datos procedentes de casi 90 series de ensayos efectuados por unos 60 científicos participantes. El rendimiento de cuatro tipos de ensayos se estimó suficiente para considerarlos como posibles pruebas complementarias del ensayo de salmonelas. Incluyeron las pruebas para la determinación de aberraciones cromosómicas, mutaciones génicas y transformaciones neoplásicas en células de mamífero en cultivo, y un ensayo para determinar la aneuploidia en levaduras. Con la excepción del ensayo de aberraciones cromosómicas, resultó evidente que los protocolos utilizados en general para esas pruebas exigían evaluación adicional antes de poder considerarlos plenamente aceptables.

La principal conclusión del estudio CSSTT/1 sobre las pruebas *in vitro* fue que el empleo de los ensayos de aberraciones cromosómicas en asociación con la prueba de mutación de salmonelas podía resultar un detector primario eficaz para posibles sustancias carcinógenas nuevas.

En el estudio IPESTTC, siete de las catorce sustancias no carcinógenas presuntas dieron resultados positivos en muchas de las pruebas *in vitro*. Los limitados datos de pruebas *in vivo* disponibles procedentes de ese estudio permiten pensar que esas siete sustancias químicas eran inactivas en las pruebas a corto plazo *in vivo*. En dos pares de sustancias carcinógenas/no carcinógenas de IPESTTC (benzo[a]pireno/pireno (BP/PIR) y 2-acetilamino-fluoreno/4-acetilamino-fluoreno (2AAF/4AAF), las sustancias no carcinógenas proporcionaron buenos ejemplos de tales respuestas diferentes, de modo que se seleccion-aron esos pares de sustancias químicas para la parte *in vivo* del estudio en colaboración (CSSTT/2). Sin embargo, hubo una fuerte duda respecto a la presunta falta de cancerogenicidad del 4AAF, y una parte crucial del estudio fue el comienzo de bioensayos de cancerogenicidad a largo plazo del 2AAF y el 4AAF en ratas.

Por consiguiente, el objetivo del estudio CSSTT/2 fue producir un abarcante perfil de datos procedentes de una amplia gama de pruebas *in vivo* a corto plazo, como medio de conocer el mecanismo por el que los distintos puntos finales genéticos de los tejidos destinatarios fundamentales responden a sustancias químicas definidas como genotóxicas *in vitro*. La meta final consistía en identificar qué ensayos *in vivo* podrían usarse para determinar la actividad in vivo de los productos genotóxicos probados.

Participaron en el proyecto de pruebas *in vivo* 97 investigadores de 16 países y se presentaron datos de unas cincuenta técnicas *in vivo* distintas. Los resultados se evaluaron en una reunión de investigadores celebrada en Cap d'Agde (Francia) en mayo de 1985. Se preparó una serie de informes que comprendían una evaluación de cada grupo de ensayos, informes resumidos sobre los ensayos en células germinales y las pruebas hepáticas específicas, e informes resumidos sobre la base total de datos correspondiente a cada par de sustancias químicas. Después se preparó un examen general de todo el estudio *in vivo* listo para la publicación final.

Sólo una pequeña proporción de los ensayos representados en el estudio CSSTT/2 satisficieron los criterios que

Resumen

definen una prueba *in vivo* a corto plazo aceptable. Sin embargo, los ensayos incluidos en el estudio no se limitaron a los que podían cumplir con más probabilidad los criterios. Así, aunque los datos procedían de ensayos que no estaban destinados fundamentalmente a identificar la genotoxicidad *in vivo*, proporcionaron información sobre un amplio espectro de efectos biológicos de las cuatro sustancias químicas. La mayoría de los ensayos en células sométicas *in vivo* para determinar la genotoxicidad discriminaron entre las sustancias carcinógenas/no carcinógenas de los dos pares, aunque en algunos casos se detectó una actividad débil en las pruebas con sustancias no carcinógenas, en particular con el 4AAF. La insensibilidad de algunos ensayos a uno u otro de los dos pares de productos químicos apoya el concepto de que deben obtenerse datos *in vivo* negativos en dos ensayos por lo menos en diferentes tejidos antes de que pueda aceptarse que una sustancia química carece de genotoxicidad *in vivo*.

Se confirmó que la prueba de micronúcleos de médula ósea de ratón es un ensayo potente, sensible y reproducible, que se recomienda para las pruebas *in vivo* primarias de las sustancias genotóxicas *in vitro*. El rendimiento general del ensayo en células hepáticas de rata para la síntesis no programada de ADN permite pensar que puede ser complementario de la prueba de micronúcleos, aunque requieren investigación adicional ciertos aspectos de sensibilidad y selectividad de ese ensayo. Se llegó a la conclusión de que ciertos ensayos ampliamente sustentados, que incluyen los de mutagenicidad por orina y mediada por el huésped y las pruebas que utilizan la mosca drosófila, son inapropiados para la evaluación de riesgos.

Los resultados del estudio CSSTT/2 confirmaron que las pruebas *in vivo* a corto plazo tienen que desempeñar una función crucial en la evaluación de los riesgos y que esa función consiste en identificar los productos químicos que, una vez demostrada la genotoxicidad *in vitro*, son activos *in vivo* y tienen así mayores probabilidades de presentar un riesgo de cancerogenicidad o mutagenicidad para los mamíferos, incluido el hombre.

www.ingramcontent.com/pod-product-compliance
Ingram Content Group UK Ltd.
Pitfield, Milton Keynes, MK11 3LW, UK
UKHW021308180426
11947UKWH00015B/1099